I0118999

Health and Fitness in the Older Adult

By Esther Winterfeldt & Debbie Miller

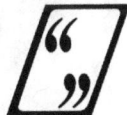

NEW FORUMS

NEW FORUMS PRESS INC.

Published in the United States of America
by New Forums Press, Inc.1018 S. Lewis St.
Stillwater, OK 74074
www.newforums.com

Copyright © 2018 by New Forums Press, Inc.

All rights reserved. No part of this publication may be reproduced or transmitted in any form or by any means, electronic or mechanical, including photocopy, or any information storage or retrieval system, without permission in writing from the publisher.

Library of Congress Cataloging-in-Publication Data Pending

This book may be ordered in bulk quantities at discount from New Forums Press, Inc., P.O. Box 876, Stillwater, OK 74076 [Federal I.D. No. 73 1123239]. Printed in the United States of America.

ISBN 10: 1-58107-315-1
ISBN 13: 978-1-58107-315-7

Contents

Introduction

Health and fitness throughout life are goals that people universally strive for and they become even more important with age. Among the many lifestyle factors that influence how well one ages and remains healthy, nutrition and physical activity lead the list. Because of the importance of these two factors in successful aging, we have concentrated on them in this book by showing how they are practiced at a leading retirement center in Oklahoma. By describing actions and procedures followed at Spanish Cove in Yukon, we encourage others to consider similar ideas to promote health and fitness for older persons living independently or with assistance. We realize that other psychological and social factors are also important for health and well-being among older adults and these are also discussed in the book although in a briefer way. Testing for mental health is usually included as a part of the overall fitness testing and is discussed in some detail in one chapter. Our hope is that all older persons have the information and the opportunities needed for lifestyles that enhance their overall health and fitness for productive and enjoyable later years.

Spanish Cove Retirement Village, located in Yukon, Oklahoma, has a record of outstanding service for retirees for over 40 years. Offering all levels of care, from independent living to nursing care, the administration encourages practices that help residents live healthy lives as long as possible. A variety of physical activities, nutritious food, and educational and recreational activities are offered.

The Authors

Esther Winterfeldt is a retired Regents Professor of Nutrition and Dietetics and department head at Oklahoma State University and is a resident of Spanish Cove. With the B.S. and M.S. from Oklahoma State and the PhD from Ohio State University, she has practiced in hospital dietetics at the University of

Chicago Hospitals and was director of dietetics at the Ohio State University Hospitals. Active in the dietetics profession, she served as president of the American Dietetic Association. She spent 28 years in higher education at Oklahoma State, Auburn University and the University of Texas-Houston. She is the author of "Aging in Good Health", "Aging in Good Mental Health", "Be Healthy: Prevent Disease" and "Our Food and Its Origins".

Debbie Miller is the director of wellness and resident relations at Spanish Cove—a position she has held for over twenty five years. She holds a B.A. degree in Communications and Public Relations from the University of Central Oklahoma. She is a certified Personal Trainer and certified Fitness Specialist for Older Adults from the Cooper Institute in Dallas, Texas. She is, further, a Master Trainer of Tai Chi for better balance as well as trained in Yoga.

The authors extend recognition and appreciation to the University of Central Oklahoma Nursing students and their faculty instructor, Dr. Rollins, for conducting the fitness testing of residents and for their enthusiastic support of the programs at Spanish Cove.

Preface

Conquistador Ponce de Leon began his search for the fountain of youth over 500 years ago. The fountain was never found but his desire to make an older body become younger still exists as strong as ever today.

Somewhere down the line we realized hopes for life extension were better placed in factors other than a magic fountain. Devotion to public health and medicine brought great success to extending life. The average lifespan during Ponce's time was between 30-40 years. Today, average life expectancy in our nation is 78 years and climbing.

Though aging has been our reward, we have not perfected it. There remains a wide gap between quantity and quality of life. Far too many seniors spend golden years with chronic health problems or other debilitating challenges. Sadly, many of these problems resulted from bad choices or habits. Ben Franklin said it well when he penned "an ounce of prevention is worth a pound of cure."

Whatever your age or condition, enjoying life to the fullest is most likely your heart's desire. While you cannot make an older body chronologically younger, it is quite possible to make an aging body more healthy.

This book provides practical insight and applications for successful aging. Many of the innovations and strategies presented within its pages have been utilized at the Spanish Cove Retirement Village for many years. It is our goal at Spanish Cove to promote health and fitness among residents in order to maximize an independent lifestyle. Use of these strategies have enabled our community to attain an average level of 87.5 years before independence is lost and either assisted living or nursing care is needed.

The extension of life will always be a long sought treasure for earth's inhabitants. Yet most would agree there is no advantage to living longer unless you can enjoy it. Quality of life is precious to us and the primary ingredient for living longer better.

Ironically, Ponce de Leon, although coming up empty in his quest, was on a good track for longevity. The physical exercise gained as result of his journey pointed him in the right direction. Had it not been for a poisoned arrow striking him on his second journey, Ponce may have lived to be a very old man.

> Don Blose
> CEO/Executive Administrator
> Spanish Cove Retirement Village

Abraham Lincoln stated, "And in the end, it's not the years in your life that count. It's the life in your years. Little did he know that decades later older adults would be defining the life in their years by changing the way they age. Older adults can have both years and life! No longer should we consider aging as a gradual decline in functional ability. That is not normal aging. In fact, less than 30% of aging is determined by genetics. Over 70% is determined by one's lifestyle. It is important for all individuals to realize that growing older does not have to mean giving up anything: activities, driving, or sport s. It's all in what we know, what we do, and how we do it.

This book uncovers the path for successful aging. Knowledge is power, and in this case, this knowledge is a powerful tool to ensure that you have quality of life until the end of your life.

Mary Brinkley
Executive Director, Leading Age OK

caremerge

The DIMENSIONS

OF WELLNESS

1 Spiritual
Establishing peace and harmony in our lives by finding a connection to our inner values which helps give more meaning to our days.

2 Emotional
Understanding ourselves and coping with the challenges life can bring. Being able to acknowledge and share feelings in a productive manner.

3 Purposeful
The desire to feel a greater sense of meaning and purpose with activities that lead to agreement between personal values and actions.

4 Vocational
Staying connected or giving back to our community with skills from past careers through knowledge sharing, consulting or volunteering.

5 Intellectual
Finding ways to expand our skills and knowledge by learning new concepts, improving existing skills and seeking challenges in pursuit of lifelong learning.

Social 6
Relating to and connecting with other people. Our ability to establish and maintain positive relationships with family, friends and co-workers.

Physical 7
Maintaining a healthy quality of life with activities that allow us to get through our daily activities without undue fatigue or physical stress.

Nutritional 8
The importance of maintaining a healthy diet, and rejuvenating our bodies through diet and food choices.

Health Services 9
Routine medical exams, immunizations and screenings to maintain our physical and mental health.

Environmental 10
Staying active by getting outdoors for activities. Learning about and making a positive impact on our environment.

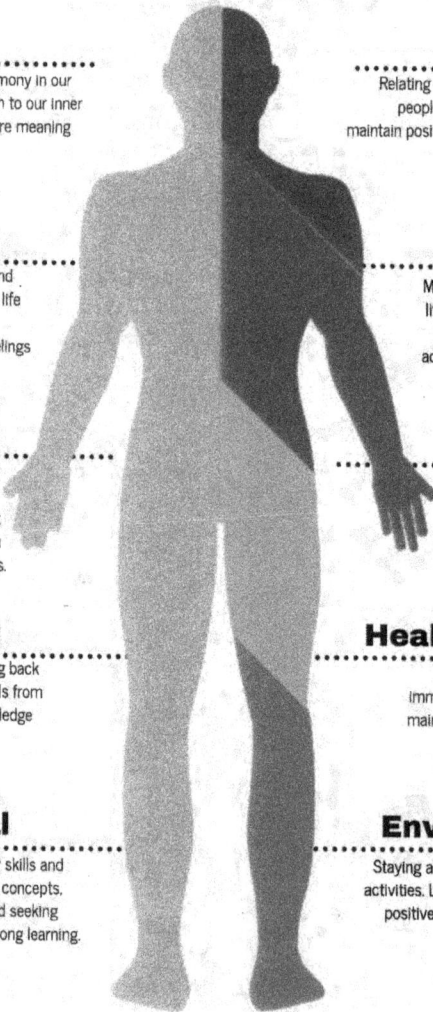

Contact us:
T: (888)996-6993
W: caremerge.com
E: sales@caremerge.com

Chapter 1
The Normal Aging Process

Age is just a number, but a number that brings challenges in daily living habits and in overall health. We slow down, we become aware of aches and pains not there before and that its harder to do some of the things we've always enjoyed. We have to think longer to recall names and phone numbers and where we left the keys.

People age at different rates and in different ways. No one has yet been able to identify the specific point at which we may be considered old. The process, however, comes about with natural changes in cells that cause a slow-down or alteration in their capacity to function in the usual way. Some researchers say that our peak functioning occurs at about age 30 and this may mean another 50-60 years to continue to live and function. How well we function during those later years depends in great part on how well we follow healthful practices and good living habits.

Mayo Clinic researchers define the aging process as "the gradual accumulation of minor body injuries or degeneration often associated with a gradual decrease in functional capacity that affects all humans to a greater or lesser degree after middle age." (1)

Physical Changes in the Aging Body

Physical changes vary among individuals and while some may appear in early middle age, others appear later. However, most people can expect to see some degree of change in the following physical systems of the body.

1. Cardiovascular system. The heart rate slows and the heart increases in size. Blood vessels tend to stiffen with resulting high blood pressure. It is estimated that more than half of those over 60 have hypertension due to the changes in blood vessels.

2. Bones, joints and muscles. The bones shrink in size and density causing a loss in height and, often, easily broken bones. Muscles stiffen leading to less coordination and balance. Degeneration of joints is common leading to arthritis and difficulty in movement.

3. Digestive system changes, especially constipation, often occur as well as dyspepsia and other stomach disorders.

4. Bladder and urinary tract. The bladder tends to shrink leading to urgency and incontinence.

5. Eyes and ears. The eyes become sensitive to glare and lose light adaptation. There is often difficulty hearing high frequencies and other hearing problems.

6. Teeth and gums. Receding gums are common and medications may cause dry mouth. Poor dental health may interfere with chewing and enjoyment of food.

7. Taste and smell. The two are interconnected so that changes in either may lead to interference with food selection leading to excessive body weight and malnutrition.

8. Skin. The skin thins and becomes less elastic. The loss of fatty tissue under the skin is the main cause. Skin changes can lead to easy bruises, wrinkles, age spots and small growths.

9. Weight. When muscle mass decreases, fat often increases. Fat burns less calories and may therefore lead to weight accumulation.

Other Changes in Aging

Mental changes. Momentary lapses in memory as in remembering familiar words or names are common. There is also less ability for multi-tasking and, usually, a longer period of time to learn new things or to concentrate. Memory loss leading to some form or degree of dementia or even Alzheimer's may occur. There are a number of warning signs that signify that some change in mental function may be occurring, such as changes in mood, energy level or appetite; difficulty sleeping; difficulty concentrating and feeling restless or on edge or increased worry or stress. (2)

Immune System Changes. A healthy immune system defends against infection and destroys foreign cells. However changes in immunity are common in aging and as a result older adults have an increased risk of susceptibility to infections, malignancy and autoimmune disorders. (3) Such declines in immune function may lead to less ability to combat viruses, bacteria and other infections and cause upper respiratory and urinary tract infections as well as pressure sores and foodborne illnesses.

Nervous System Changes. With advancing age the brain and nervous system go through natural variations. The number of nerve cells and the total weight of the brain and spinal cord are reduced and message-processing time increases. Such changes can in turn contribute to reduced food intake and affect gastrointestinal function in the digestion of food and absorption of nutrients. (4)

Endocrine System Changes. The aging process is characterized by many changes in hormone production and activity. These changes affect many of the body's metabolic functions and can lead to alterations in energy and nutrient metabolism. Thyroid hormones and estrogen levels decrease with age and both affect bone metabolism. Age-related changes in hormones also play a role in the development of frailty and sarcopenia. (5)

Hematologic Changes. Anemia is a common health problem in older adults. A rate of 20 percent prevalence among persons older than age 85 has been observed and almost ten percent of the entire older adult population suffer from some type of anemia. (6) Anemia is associated with functional impairment and physical decline with decreased quality of life.

The Effect of Changes in the Older Adult

Are all these changes inevitable? As indicated, people do differ in the degree to which they may develop these physical and mental changes. The aging process cannot be stopped but the severity and impact may be lessened through the adoption of healthy lifestyles and health-related choices we make even after the aging process is underway. Researchers continue to find new clues that may make it possible in the future to delay and/or lessen the changes that occur. The National Institute on Aging is a leading agency undertaking this research and also for funding other research by institutions and universities. The Institute provides information to the public regarding genetic, clinical, behavioral, social and economic aspects of aging through both in-house and externally funded research. The Office of Nutrition and Health Promotion in the Administration on Aging conducts many programs aiding older citizens. Such programs include behavioral health information, chronic disease self-management programs and disease prevention and health promotion services. (7) The expanding number of older citizens means that both education and access to health promotion programs will be increasingly needed.

Theories of Aging

Among the many theories on aging that have been put forth, they appear to fall into two main categories: *programmed and damage or error. (8)* The programmed theory is based on the implication that aging follows a biological timetable while the damage theory emphasizes environmental impacts that lead to a build-up of damage at various levels that lead to aging. The programmed theory includes sub-categories: *programmed longevity* which refers to the switching on and off genes with eventual deficits and the *endocrine* theory that holds that hormones control the pace of aging, and, finally, the *immunological* theory that refers to the decline of the immune system over time, leading to aging and death.

The damage theory emphasizes the wear and tear, the rate of living, protein cross-linking, free radicals that damage cells, and DNA damage. Restricting calories in lab animals has been shown to prolong their life although it is not known if the same applies to humans. The gradual decrease in telomere length on the ends of chromosomes is also believed to cause changes that lead to aging. (9)

What can we do to age in the best possible way? While genetics is a sizeable factor in aging, we now know that lifestyle practices may be even more important in the aging process. This means we have considerable control over how and when we age. The lifestyle factors thought to be primarily involved in the aging process are discussed in the next chapter.

Due to our modern-day marketing practices and media coverage, many practices and products touted as "anti-aging" are at times proposed but many are questionable. Examples are herbal supplements, specific vitamin and mineral supplements, hormones, wrinkle removers, plastic surgery, anti-obesity surgery and others. "Beware of health scams" is one of the recommendations from the Baltimore Longitudinal Study on Aging. (10) This is an important reminder both for maintaining health and preventing chronic disease and for delaying the changes of aging for as long as possible.

Summary

Physical, mental and other biological changes occur as people age. The effects of these changes may be far-reaching and lead to disabilities and increasing frailty. Realizing that many changes are gene-related but are affected to a greater degree by lifestyle factors means we have some degree of control over how and when we age and our state of health.

References

1. "Aging—what to expect". Mayo Clinic Newsletter. January 1, 2013.

2. Older adults-and-mental health. www.nimih.nih.gov

3. Simpson RJ, Guy K. Coupling aging immunity with a sedentary lifestyle: has the damage already been done? Gerontology 2010;56(5):449-458.

4. How the nervous system changes as you age. Remedy Health Media. New York. www.heath-central.com/Alzheimer's/stages

5. Morley JE, Mahlmston TK. Frailty, sarcopenia and hormones. Endocrin Metab Clin North Am 2013;42(2):391-405.

6. Guralnik JM, Eisenstaent RS, Ferrell L, Klein HI, Woodman RD. Prevalence of anemia in persons 65 years and older in the United States: evidence for a high rate of unexplained anemia. Blood 2004;104:2263-2268.

7. www.oaa.dhhs.gov

8. Kunlin J. Modern biological theories of aging. Aging Dis 2010;1(2):72-74.

9. Valdes AM, Deary IJ, Gardner J et al. Leukocyte telomere length is associated with cognitive performance in healthy women. Neurobiology of Aging 2010;31:986-992.

10. Shock NW, et al. Normal human aging: the Baltimore Longitudinal Study on Aging. www.blsa.gov

Chapter 2

Lifestyle Factors in Aging

"Successful aging" is a universal goal. We will age—regardless of what our life is like up to the point at which we recognize we are old. There is no one definition of aging—it is different for everyone and there is no agreement as to the age at which it begins. Some are old at age 50; others are essentially young at age 80. The age of 65 set by the Social Security Act as the retirement age in the 1930's was an arbitrary number designated by the government. It was based on the life expectancy of about 67 at the time. It fits for some but not for others who have another 20 to 30 years of life. Those later years can be productive, useful years with good health and a lifestyle that allows persons to remain active and engaged.

Health and aging are outcomes of both genetic and environmental conditions. It is fortunate that living styles appear to be of even greater importance than what we inherit. By a process termed "epigenetics", it is now known that lifestyle activities can even impact the genes for better or worse.

Successful aging simply means aging well. The three main components of successful aging, according to a leading gerontologist are: avoiding disease and disability, maintaining physical and mental function, and continuing engagement in life. (1) Specific activities that meet these criteria are discussed further.

Exercise and Physical Activity

The role of physical activity cannot be over-emphasized in how we age. The National Institute on Aging defines physical activities as those that get the body moving such as gardening, walking the dog, raking leaves, taking the stairs instead of the elevator. Exercise in the form of physical activity that is structured and repetitive such as weight training, tai chi, stretch and strength and yoga are excellent choices.

The benefits of physical activity are reduced risk of developing some diseases and disabilities such as arthritis, heart disease, diabetes and hypertension. Balance problems and difficulty in walking can also be helped by exercise. Exercise is also recommended as an antidepressant and a way of reducing the risk of dementia. The amount and kinds of exercise recommended for older adults are discussed in more detail in Chapters 4 and 5.

Nutrition

Throughout life we make choices about what we eat. There may be many reasons but the accumulated effect of the choices has a direct relationship to aging well. The healthful food choices that align with recommendations from research enable us to realize the following benefits:

- To enable growth and development
- For the production of energy for body functions
- To stave off chronic disease through nutrient reactions
- To strengthen the immune system for disease resistance
- To maintain optimum body weight and weight changes over time
- To keep bones strong and resistant to thinning
- To maintain mental function
- To help genes function for the best health benefits
- To build and preserve muscular strength

The role of nutrition as related to overall health is expanded in Chapter 8 and with discussion of the Dietary Guidelines in Chapter 10.

Sleep

It has long been recognized that sleep is somehow essential to health and research within the past 20 years has now begun to tell us why. Sleep deprivation negatively affects brain function including memory, emotions and regulation of appetite. During sleep, the immune system produces higher levels of antibodies that ward off disease. Hormone levels are affected without enough sleep—primarily insulin and leptin which control diabetes and body weight. Depression is another outcome of poor or inadequate sleep. The clearance of waste products such as beta amyloid, which is implicated in Alzheimer's disease, has also been shown to occur during sleep.

Seven to eight hours of sleep is the recommended amount. An observation about the need for sleep is pointed out in the following: "the result of studies looking at the role of sleep in hormonal, immunological and memory functions suggests that if you do not get enough you could—besides being very tired—wind up sickly, overweight, forgetful and very blue. " (2)

Stress. Everyone experiences stress at times. It is how the body and brain respond to situations caused by anxiety or un-certainty. Stress may be an only once-in-a-while occurrence and is handled without causing any long-term effects. The body's reaction to stress leads to the production of adrenal hormones—cortisol, adrenaline and norepinephrine. Adrenaline and norepi-nephrine cause a rise in energy and incite the "fight or flight" syndrome.

There are different types of stress and all carry physical and mental health risks. (3) Stress can at times motivate people to prepare or perform or even to face a life-saving situation. The pulse quickens, the breath is faster, the muscles tense and the brain uses more oxygen and becomes more active.

Long-term stress can lead to suppression of the immune sys-tem, interfere with digestion and sleep and upset the reproductive system. People under chronic stress are prone to more frequent and severe viral infections. In time, serious health problems may result such as heart disease, hypertension, diabetes and others as well as mental health problems like dementia.

Managing stress includes being aware of physical signs such as difficulty sleeping, increased use of alcohol or other substances, being easily angered, feeling depressed and having low energy. Getting exercise, trying a relaxing activity and setting goals and priorities with timelines and positive outcomes are all helpful techniques to overcome stress.

Mental Health

The National Institute of Mental Health provides a lengthy list of mental disorders and ongoing research into each of the disorders. (4) Notable among these are conditions that may be more prevalent among older adults such as anxiety, bipolar disorder or substance abuse. The ultimate chronic mental disorder—Alzheimer's—as well as other dementias, are most common among older adults. A relatively high proportion of those 85 or above are considered to be at risk. Steps that can be taken to help prevent and treat various types of mental disorders are discussed in Chapter 6.

Social Contacts. It is well established that people of all ages need social connections in order to maintain overall health. The companionship of sharing meals and special occasions leads to greater enjoyment of the meal and a better food intake. Interactions with family and friends maintains mental health and can help overcome depression and loneliness. Joining groups, participating in continuing educational activities, card games and other events of particular interest are all beneficial in maintaining a healthy mind-body connection.

Substance Abuse

Smoking, excessive use of alcohol or medications and drugs are all detrimental to health at any age but especially in later ages. Countless research studies have shown adverse physical and mental effects: cancer, heart disease, liver disease and malnutrition. In addition, there is a greater tendency to contract other diseases due to a weakened immune system. Alcohol, in moderation, may have some beneficial effect, primarily in heart disease. But in amounts greater than one drink a day for women and two for men there can be adverse effects. (5)

Summary

The overall health of the older adult is an outcome of both genetic and environmental factors. Important activities that affect the aging process such as exercise, nutrition, stress, and substance abuse may be of more significance over time than inherited traits.

References

1. Moody HR, Sasser JR. *Aging: Concepts and Controversies.* 7th ed. Sage Publisher, Los Angeles, 2012.

2. Stickgold R. Sleep on it! Scientific American 2015;313(4):52-57.

3. Five Things You Should Know about Stress. www.nimha.gov/health publications

4. www.nimh.gov/healthtopics.for older adults

5. www.nimh/gov.healthtopics.olderadults

6. Dietary Guidelines for Americans. 2015-2020. www.cnnp.usda.gov

Chapter 3

The Relationship Between Health and Fitness

Hippocrates advised several centuries ago: "let food be your medicine". This was well before any knowledge of the role of nutrition and other lifestyle practices was available to medical practitioners. It is now known that most diseases that occur during the later stages of life have developed over extended periods of time and that the causes may be due to a combination of genetic and environmental factors. The population is growing older and, beginning at about age 65, two-thirds of the chronic disabling conditions occur. The leading causes of death—cardiovascular conditions, cancer, diabetes and lung disease—account for the greatest health care costs and need for care by this segment of the population. According to the "Healthy People 2010-2020" report, health disparities such as health literacy or inability to read instructions and understand prescribed treatments, being disabled, those living in rural areas, race, ethnicity, income and education are all factors that may impact health and health care. (1)

Because many of the organ systems in the body become less active during aging, our overall resistance to disease is also lessened. The defense system is compromised when immunological factors are lessened. Defining fitness as the suitability or adaptation to body changes and its ability to maintain a state of health, we can look further at the physical and mental factors associated with good health.

The lifestyle factors pointed out in Chapter 2 are, first and foremost, applicable to maintaining a state of fitness and are under our control. All have been extensively researched and shown to help promote health and to delay or prevent the onset of disease. The relationship between health and fitness is reciprocal—health is affected if fitness is lacking and fitness is seldom seen in the absence of physical and mental health. The interplay between the

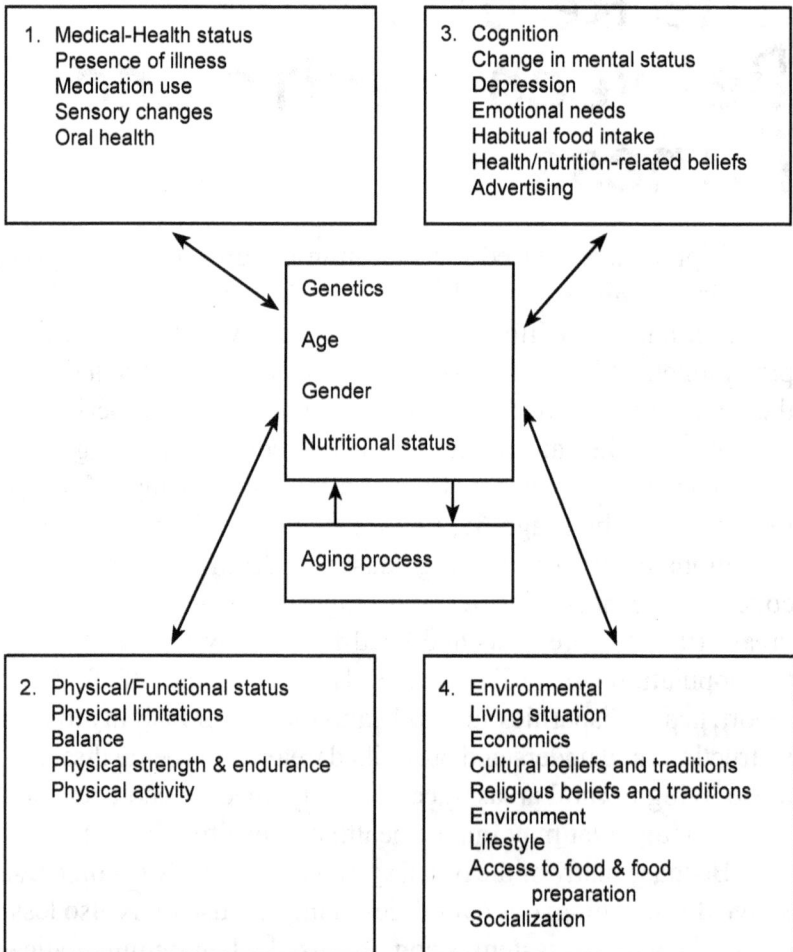

Figure 1. Factors in Health-Related Quality of Life and Aging
(Adapted from: Position of the Academy of Nutrition and Dietetics: Food for the older adult, promoting health and wellness. J Acad Nutr Acad 2012;112(8):1255-1277).

many factors that work together to influence aging and overall health is shown in Figure 1.

Frailty in Older Persons

"I don't feel like myself" is a comment often heard when something is lacking such as a feeling of inability to do the things we need or want to do. Frailty may be one of the major causes for this feeling as it is a condition that affects both physical and mental capability. It is defined as a syndrome involving reduced functional reserve, impaired mobility, decreased strength and endurance, increased feelings of exhaustion, inactivity and decreased quality of life. It is strongly associated with unintentional weight loss, muscle wasting (sarcopenia) and malnutrition. (2) The older frail are at increased risk of functional limitations, disability, dependency and the need for long-term care.

Frailty typically develops slowly over time. Factors thought to contribute to the onset include genetics, epigenetics, environment (nutrition and physical activity), chronic inflammation and hormonal changes. Obviously, this is not a condition that can be easily reversed but taking steps such as regular exercise and good nutritional intake can play a large role. And the earlier in life the steps are taken, the better the chances of maintaining health longer and avoiding frailty.

Frailty and malnutrition often coexist among older adults so that nutritional screening is important when persons have been identified as being at risk for these conditions. Several screening instruments are available to be used and others are described in chapter 8. (3)

A consensus group from six major international European and U.S. societies in 2013 found that physical frailty can potentially be prevented or treated with actions such as exercise, protein-calorie supplementation, vitamin D, and fewer pharmaceuticals. Studies about the efficacy of dietary treatments have shown that optimum dietary intakes can lead to improved strength, walking speed and nutritional status in a majority of frail older adults. Increasing protein and vitamin D intake seem to be among the most effective.

Disability is described as a decline in physical ability or mental capacity leading to the inability to perform the usual activities of daily living without great difficulty. Being disabled is not a normal part of aging. The relationship between frailty and disability may be close and may mean hardship on families and assistance personnel as well as continued decline of the older person.

Quality of Life

"Quality of life" may be simply described as the ability to enjoy normal life activities. It does not automatically decline with age although older adults are more often at risk of experiencing

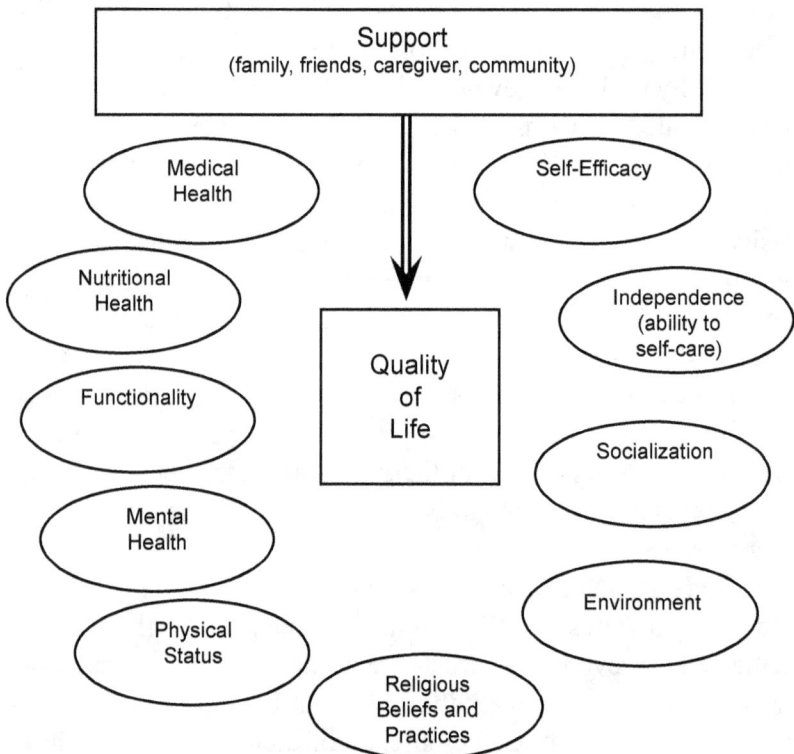

Figure 2. Factors that Influence Quality of Life
(Adapted from Position Paper of the American Dietetic Association: Nutrition across the spectrum of aging. J Am Diet Assoc 2005; 105(4):616-633.)

this decline. There are several dimensions to the quality of life: physical, emotional, psychological and spiritual. The many factors that influence the quality of life are shown in Figure 2.

According to the Centers for Disease Control (CDC), measures of health outcomes are the basis of saving lives and for improving the quality of lives. They refer to a "Health-related Quality of Life" (HRQOL) as a way to being together social, mental, and medical aspects of life. (4) The HRQOL is often used to measure the effects of chronic disease, to better understand how an illness interferes with personal day-to-day life and to measure the effects of numerous disorders and short-and long-term disabilities and disease. Questionnaires have been designed to measure the HTQOL for individuals and for communities. They are used by the CDC and in the National Health and Nutrition Examination Surveys (NHANES), conducted by areas of the U.S. to determine overall nutritional health. (5)

The importance of nutrition in healthy aging and in reducing the financial and societal burden of the increasing aging population, is shown in a recent national report: "Nutritional Considerations for Healthy Aging and Reduction in Age-Related Chronic Disease". (6) The report indicates that a large portion of the population will be vulnerable to nutritional frailty, characterized by significant weight-loss and loss of muscle mass and strength---or a loss of physiologic reserves. There will be even greater need to identify specific nutrient needs, biomarkers to understand the impact of advancing age on protein requirements, skeletal muscle turnover and how BMI (Body Mass Index) guidelines are best applied.

A large-scale study in Australia of 1305 persons over 55 years of age, followed for five and ten years, found that the higher the diet quality, the better the quality of life and functional ability. (7) There was a positive association between diet quality and the ability to perform instrumental activities of daily living (IADL) and concurrence with U.S. studies showing an association between higher scores on the Healthy Eating Index and IADL.

Successful aging and overall fitness are desired outcomes of the aging process for all. The many factors that enter into the quality of life largely determine the extent to which these outcomes are realized.

Energy

A decline in energy need occurs with age. This is due to a gradual decrease in the body's three types of energy uses. The energy need for basal metabolism or basal metabolic rate (BMR) is the largest at 60-75%. These are the need for internal, involuntary functions such as heart beat, respiration, blood flow etc. Physical activity accounts for 15-35% of energy need while the thermic effect of foods (TEF) needs less than 10%. The TEf represents the energy needed to digest and metabolize food. The reason for the BMR decrease is primarily reduction in the lean body mass while activity tends to decrease for whatever reason. It is estimated that there is about 10% less energy needed each decade of life.

Although there are individual differences-- in general, after about age 60, the boy weight decreases due to, usually, a more sedentary lifestyle with a resulting loss of lean body mass or sarcopenia. This can lead to increased disability and functional dependence. A loss of bone and muscle leads to reduced strength.

Even though less energy is needed overall, the body's nutrient needs remain the same. Therefore, if appetite and food intake remain the same, overweight will be the result. In a further chapter, the consequences of both overweight and underweight are discussed.

Fitness Age

A Scandinavian study recently reported a way to assess aerobic fitness by estimating a "fitness age". (8) It is based on oxygen intake without a treadmill test. In the study, participants in an "active leisure" group were at a 30% lower risk for all-cause mortality and 27% less likely to suffer a first-time cardiovascular event. Active-leisure seniors were also metabolically healthier. Men and women who were active in their free time tended to have a smaller waist circumference, higher HDL cholesterol levels and lower triglycerides. Among men, active leisure was associated with better insulin and blood sugar levels although it was not associated with lower blood pressure.

Summary

Health and fitness among older adults are outcomes of both genetic and lifestyle factors. Frailty may develop due to a variety of reasons, however consistent exercise and a good nutritional intake help preserve functionality longer. The quality of life is directly affected by overall fitness and the ability to remain active and in good health.

References

1. www.healthypeople.nih.gov
2. Firmhaber GC, Kolasa KM. "I don't feel like myself". Treating frailty in the elderly with diet. Nutrition Today 2016;15(6):281-288.
3. LaurC, Keller H. Making the Case for Nutrition Screening in Older Adults in Primary Care. Nutrition Today 2017;52(30;129-136.
4. Morley JE, Vellos B, Kan GA, et al. Frailty concerns: A call to action. J Am Med Assoc 2013;14(6):392-397.
5. www.cdc.gov. HRQOL Concepts.
6. Bernstein M, Munoz N. *Nutrition for the Older Adult.* 2nd ed. Jones and Bartlett, Publisher, Burlington, MA.
7. "Nutritional Considerations for healthy aging, reduction in age-related chronic diseases". www.science daily.com/releases. Source: Tufts U. 2017.
8. What's Your "Fitness Age"? Tufts U. Health and Nutrition newsletter. 2014;31(12)"1.

Chapter 4
Keys to Gaining and Maintaining Fitness

With age, being active maintains and even increases physical and mental abilities while inactivity magnifies age-related changes. Physical health is the continual growth of physical function and includes actions that limit or prevent disease and disability. Cardiovascular activity, strength, balance, flexibility, nutrition, sleep and preventive health screenings are all keys to physical health. Being active in these areas provides numerous health benefits in older adults and may help lower the risk for heart disease, stroke, diabetes, osteoporosis, depression, cancer and Alzheimer's disease.

Activity through exercise can diminish the risk of falls, improve mental health and slow the aging process. Regular physical activity is associated with decreased early mortality and age-related morbidity in older adults. Unfortunately, up to 75 percent of older Americans are insufficiently active to achieve these and other health benefits. (1) Few contraindications to exercise exist and people of all ages can benefit from additional physical activity. The sedentary person may experience more severe health problems than the more active, exercising individual.

Physical Activity: Kind and Amount

The exercise prescription most often recommended for older adults consists of four key components: cardiovascular (aerobic) exercise, strength training, flexibility and balance training. Each of these components are described in the following paragraphs.

Cardiovascular or Aerobic Exercise

The goal of aerobic exercise is to increase cardiovascular endurance. The Centers for Disease Control defines aerobic exercise as any action that increases the respiratory and heart rate above normal resting rate, sustained for at least ten minutes. Generally healthy adults over the age of 65 should aim for 150 minutes of moderately intensive activity a week. (2) One of the best forms of cardiovascular exercise is walking. It is safe, easy to do, requires no equipment and has numerous benefits. It is important for the older adult to walk in order to remain active and independent. Beginning walkers should start slowly by walking short distances and gradually increasing the distance. Walking at a comfortable pace and focusing on good posture gives the best results.

Research has shown that walking 6 to 9 miles a week can prevent brain shrinkage and memory loss. According to the American Academy of Neurology, older adults who walked this much had more gray matter in their brains nine years after the start of the study than people who walked less. (3)

Warm-up exercises for five to ten minutes before starting an exercise session are important to prevent injury by increasing the heart rate and respiration and increasing body temperature which in turn warms the muscles. Regardless of the activity level, it is essential to begin slowly and build up the level of warm-up time. Warming the body before exercise also plays a big role in preventing injury. A typical warm-up may consist of stretching, a slow walk or any light activity such as any chosen cardiovascular exercise at a slower, more relaxed pace. Gentle stretches and range of motion exercises at the end of the warm-up helps increase flexibility. The warm-up usually lasts 5 to 10 minutes.

The main exercise, also called endurance training, should consist of activities that use the large muscle groups to increase heart rate for an extended period of time. Using the arms and legs vigorously will do this. Following the exercise, five to fifteen minutes of low-level cool down activities bring the heart rate down and stretch out the muscles. Cool down exercises help improve flexibility.

The level of effort put into activity is likely to agree with the effort that actual physical measurements would reveal. A way to estimate how extensively and at what level one should exercise is by using a measurement called the Borg scale. This is a colored, numerical scale showing a minimal activity level from 6 to a maximum level of 20. (4)

A. Low-Intensity Cardiovascular Exercise

This type of exercise only slightly increases the heart and breathing rate and is therefore encouraged for older adults with medical conditions that may make exercise particularly difficult or dangerous. The most popular and easy-to-do low intensity exercise is walking. Walking at a slow pace during normal activities of daily living, such as shopping, can count toward the weekly goal. Gardening and bicycling are other examples of low intensity cardiovascular exercise as is swimming or low impact water aerobics for seniors with arthritis. They place less strain on the joints and are very low impact. During this type of activity, the older adult would not be breathing hard or sweating.

B. Moderate-Intensity Cardiovascular Exercise

This type of exercise includes brisk walking, swimming, cycling, tennis, dancing and hikin. Moderate exercise uses large muscle groups and causes the body to use more oxygen. The older adult may become a little breathless or sweat but should be able to carry on a conversation during exercise. The recommended amount of time for this type exercise is the following: 30 to 60 minutes a day for 5 times a week for moderate activity or 20-60 minutes for 3 times a week for vigorous, intense exercise. Added to this are strengthening exercises 2 to 3 times a week with 10 to 15 reps according to the American College of Sports Medicine (ACSM). A more detailed version of the ACSM guidelines is included in the appendix.

C. High Intensity or Vigorous Cardiovascular Exercise

This type of exercise can be recommended and even encouraged for active, healthy older adults. Studies show that one minute of vigorous cardiovascular exercise is the equivalent of two minutes of moderate or low intensity exercise. However, there are higher risks of injury and this type of exercise puts extra stress on joints. Examples of high intensity cardiovascular exercises include running, working out on an elliptical trainer and cross country skiing.

Strength Training (Weight Lifting)

Strength training can play a critical role in helping seniors stay strong and active throughout the aging process. According to the National Institutes of Health and other research bodies, strength training is the "fountain of youth". (5) It is one of the secrets for living longer and stronger as well as helping to prevent or delay the onset of illness and disease. A decline in muscular strength contributes to increased disability, frailty and falls. This loss of muscle mass and strength is known as *sarcopenia.* Research has shown that in normal aging, after the age of 50, a person's muscular strength decreases about 15-20 percent per decade. (6)

Strength training and other exercises for seniors not only builds bone and muscle, but also help counteract the weakness and frailty that often comes with aging. There are minimal risks when strength training is done according to accepted guidelines. By increasing muscular strength and endurance due to the ability to repeat a movement over and over again, more energy is generated for other activities of daily living. According to the National Institute on Aging: "making even small changes when it comes to strength building can have big benefits, even for those people who may have already lost a lot of muscle". (7) Increases in muscle mass that may not even be visible to the eye can still make it easier to get up from chairs or climb stairs.

The principle of "overload" means that in order to improve strength and endurance, the workload needs to increase by gradually stressing a muscle by working for a longer period of time than usual or at a higher intensity level. This could mean lifting more weight or doing more repetitions.

As with cardiovascular exercise, an older adult should warm their muscles before beginning a strength training routine. A warm up might include light walking, marching in place or shoulder rolls to warm the muscles and raise the temperature. Strength training activities should include exercises for all the major muscle groups: shoulders, arms, chest, abdomen, back, hips and legs. Examples of strength training exercises include lifting free weights, using resistance bands (exerbands) or using special equipment as at a fitness center or gym.

Regular strength training should be performed two to three days a week with a rest day between sessions. Each exercise should be performed for 8 to 12 repetitions. If the older adult can lift a weight more than for 15 repetitions of an exercise, he or she can graduate to a heavier weight.

A valuable information source for strength training is the book titled "Growing Stronger—Strength Training for Older Adults". The free book is available at the Centers for Disease Control website. (www.cdc.hhs.gov)

Flexibility (Stretching) Training

With age, the muscles become shorter and can lose their elasticity. Stretching for flexibility improves the range of motion for activities of daily living and freedom of movement to do the things one needs and likes. Although flexibility and balance training are not discussed as much as cardiovascular and strength building exercises, they are a key part of physical fitness and for staying active and independent. Flexibility exercises can improve overall ease of movement, decrease stress on the joints and reduce the risk of injury. Such exercises also help improve blood flow to the muscles. According to the American College of Sports Medicine, flexibility exercise allows persons to perform everyday activities with less pain and more ease. (See ACSM guidelines, Appendix A)

Flexibility exercises should stretch all the major muscle groups to improve muscle length, flexibility and joint health.

As the saying goes: "motion is the lotion for your joints". The general rule is to perform stretching exercises two to three times a week. The older adult should begin with 5 to 10 total stretches for the upper and lower body by walking or marching in place or similar activity to warm the muscles. The stretch should be held for 30 to 60 seconds and should never cause pain, especially joint pain. However, mild discomfort or a mild pulling is normal. There are few contradictions to stretching, however, more strenuous stretching exercises are not appropriate for older adults. Mindful movement exercises like Tai Chi and Yoga focus on developing flexibility and balance with an emphasis on breathing.

Balance Training

Balance training consists of specific exercises that help build lower body muscle strength as well as improve balance. Such exercises can help prevent a fall and build confidence in walking. Some balance exercises help build leg strength while others focus on stability. The recommendation is for older adults to focus on balance training three or more days a week and can be performed daily. A fall prevention program begins with balance to help with equilibrium and the ability to quickly recover from situations when the person is unstable.

Many balance exercises are the same as lower body strengthening exercises. Examples of balance exercises include: standing from a seated position (building strength), standing on one leg (stability), tandem standing (strength and stability), and tandem walking. Practicing Tai Chi can also reduce the risk of falling by strengthening lower body muscles and training the body to balance in a variety of positions.

Exercise Benefits

For most people, the hardest part of exercise is getting started. Even if an exercise program has never been undertaken, no age is too late to start reaping the benefits. By remaining active, older persons will be able to do the things they like to do and remain independent longer. Think about fitness goals in 10-minute segments for significant benefits: ten minutes of walking, ten minutes of lifting weights, ten minutes of stretching and balance exercises. Remember too, exercising does not have to be in a gym, fitness center or class but can be followed when and where convenient. The benefits from activity are cumulative, so just several brief bouts of exercises through the day can be as good as one long exercise session. Either way, it is important to fit it into one's lifestyle in an enjoyable way to continue.

Resources for exercise benefits for seniors, the National Institute on Aging (www.nia.hhs.org) provides excellent material. For guidelines for physical activity in adults over age 65, the American College of Sports Medicine (Appendix A) is a good source.

Summary

How we age is determined in great part by lifestyle. How much we move, learn new things, connect with others and have meaning and purpose in our lives are powerful predictors of the quality and even quantity of the aging experience. By remaining active, it is possible to markedly change the aging experience by lessening sickness and impairment while extending functionality. Physical activity is safe and effective for strength, flexibility and cardiovascular health for seniors and people with different ability levels. Stretching the muscles improves range of motion and flexibility, making everyday movement easier. Cardiovascular exercise strengthens the heart and lungs and lowers the risk of developing chronic conditions including heart disease and high blood pressure as well as providing multiple other benefits. Whatever the current health condition, it can often be overcome and even reversed with exercise. The ultimate goal of successful aging is staying independent and paying attention to all aspects of life: physical, intellectual, spiritual, social and vocational.

References

1. Nied RJ, Franklin B. Promoting and prescribing exercise for the elderly. Am Family Physician. 2002;65(3).

2. Centers for Disease Control. (www.cdc.hhs.gov)

3. Walk much? University of Pittsburgh Study shows it may protect your memory down the road. Am Acad Neurology, U of Pittsburgh. 2010:10.

4. The Borg Scale of Perceived Exertion. Measuring Physical Activity Intensity. (www.cdc.hhs.gov)

5. National Institute on Aging. (www.nia.gov/health/exercise/physial activity)

6. Feland B, Meyrer JW, Schelthies SS, Fellingham GW, Meason GW. The Effect of Duration of stretching the hamstring muscle group for increasing range of motion in people aged 65 years or older. Growing Strong: Strength Training for Older Adults. Tufts University and Centers for Disease Control. 2002.

7. www.nia.hhs.gov

8. Tai chi moving for better balance. Oregon Research Center. (www.taichi moving for better balance.org)

Chapter 5
The Spanish Cove Experience in Maintaining Fitness

Our mission at Spanish Cove is to help seniors remain active and independent while experiencing life to the fullest extent possible. To this end, a number of health and fitness classes are offered for those in all areas of living: independent, assisted and nursing care. Our wellness initiative has included a program of "Living Longer, Better" for emphasis on nutrition, physical activity and social engagement. Classes offered for independent-living residents include: Stretch and Strengthen, Yoga, Line Dancing, Tai Chi, Chair Yoga, Toning and Movement, Dragon Boat paddling, Water Exercise, Water fun, a walking program and a Senior Boot Camp.

Determining an older person's current physical activity status is important when creating an exercise program and setting short and long term goals. The Physical Activity Readiness Questionnaire (PARQ) is a medical screening questionnaire commonly used. (1) The status is determined first by the person's abilities prior to beginning an exercise program, including medical clearance.

Fitness Testing

As a way to determine the effectiveness of exercise programs on the health of residents at Spanish Cove, functional fitness testing is conducted yearly. Functional fitness is defined as "having the physical capacity to perform normal everyday activities safely and independently without undue fatigue". (2) We chose to use *The Senior Fitness Test (SFT)* because it assesses physical characteristics needed for older adults to stay functionally mobile and independent. (3) The test measures functional fitness for common everyday activities, such as rising from a seat, walking, lifting, bending and stretching. The SFT also allows individual and group comparison to a national database for seven specific tests covering five indicators for successful aging. The five are: strength, balance, agility, endurance and flexibility. The SFT is safe and enjoyable for older adults while meeting scientific standards for reliability and validity.(4)

Nursing students from the University of Central Oklahoma are assigned yearly to Spanish Cove for clinical experiences which has evolved into a partnership with mutual benefit for both. As a pilot, students along with the Spanish Cove certified fitness director, conducted the first fitness test for over 100 independent-living residents. The goals were to inform the residents of their personal areas of strength and areas for needed improvement, to gain information to further identify and develop programs and activities to enhance the well-being of seniors within the community, and to seek opportunities for further research studies for Nursing students. The success of this initial pilot activity was overwhelming with positive outcomes for both Spanish Cove and the UCO Department of Nursing. As a result, the project was formalized as a research study with the potential to expand the activity beyond Spanish Cove to other senior living environments.

The Fitness testing has continued yearly. The tests are conducted over a one or two-day period. Eight testing stations are used. Each station is attended by one or two nursing students who conduct and record test results. A separate intake station collects participant demographic and anthropometric measures including height, weight and blood pressure. Upon completion of each test, individual scores are compared to national values of more than 7000 independent living adults aged 60-94. The Senior Fitness Test also allows group comparisons to a national database. The senior fitness test is safe and enjoyable for older adults while still meeting scientific standards for reliability and validity.

The tests included in the SFT database are: Chair Stand (measuring lower body strength), Arm Curl (for upper body strength), 6-minute walk (to measure aerobic endurance), 2-minute step test (for aerobic endurance), Back Scratch (measuring upper body flexibility), and the 8-foot Up-and-Go to measure agility and dynamic balance. Each of the tests are described in the following paragraphs.

The **chair stand** measures lower body strength for moving from a chair, walking and negotiating steps. It involves a count of the number of complete stands from a sitting position completed in 30 seconds. Lower body strength decreases the risk of falls by increasing muscle strength and endurance. A decline in lower body strength is a powerful predictor of the onset of disability and loss of independence. Lower body strength can be improved with exercises such as leg extensions and leg curls, squats, dancing and walking. Combining activities at varied speeds can also improve motor ability.

The **arm curl** measures upper body strength. It tests the total number of bicep curls completed in 30 seconds while holding a five pound weight (women) or eight pound weight (men). Upper body strength is important in helping opening a jar, carrying items, and performing many household chores. Both upper and lower body strength can be improved at any age by participating in regular physical activities and strength training. Better posture and helping make back and chest muscles stronger and better balanced leads to less back pain because the back muscles are able to tolerate more stress.

The **six-minute walk** is a common measurement tool used to determine basic exercise endurance and functional fitness. It is a timed walk assessment of cardiovascular or aerobic endurance. The total distance walked (measured in yards) is the score. If a person is unable to complete six minutes, the score becomes the actual distance walked. It has been shown that the walking speed of older adults in their 60s and 70s is a strong predictor of length of life. The ability to walk depends on many of the body's functions. In addition to body support, timing, power and strength, walking requires effort from the heart and lungs. Walking also requires the support of muscles, bones and joints.

The **two-minute step test** is a test that simulates climbing stairs. This step-in-place test is used for assessing the cardiovascular or aerobic levels of those who cannot walk freely. The test indicates the ability to do everyday activities, energy levels and ability to remain independent. With age, our aerobic abilities decline. In general, aerobic endurance can be improved by brisk walking or bicycling (indoors or outdoors), swimming or in an exercise class.

The **chair sit-and-reach** is a lower body and trunk flexibility test. Flexibility can be improved by stretching large muscle groups as in a stretch or yoga class. Lower boy flexibility contributes to performing mobility tasks such as getting in and out of bed or a car.

The **back scratch** is an upper body flexibility test. Tight upper body muscles can contribute to poor posture and back pain. The tightness can also affect shoulder and arm range of motion, making it difficult to perform tasks such as dressing, combing the hair, putting on a coat or reaching for a seat belt. Upper body stretches for flexibility include activities like shoulder rolls, shoulder and upper arm stretch. Shoulder range of motion also helps avoid shoulder and rotator cuff injuries.

The **8-foot-up-and-go** test is an agility and dynamic balance test. There is a gradual decline in sensory (eyes and ears), motor (muscles, tendons, joints), and cognitive(reasoning, memory) functions that affect an older adult's ability to maintain good agility and balance as they move, get up or change position. Simple exercises that focus on core strength, leg strength, agility and balance can have a tremendous effect on improving this important component of health and fitness. Exercises such as Tai Chi and dancing can do this.

A **Brief Cognitive Assessment (BCAT)** along with a Healthy senior Aging Survey, was administered to identify factors that support seniors living independently within the community. Both tests continue to be used annually. Undergraduate and graduate UCO students participate in the identification of appropriate screening tools, development of data collection instruments, administration of the tests, data analysis, and creation of future projects to work with residents and staff in the facilities to enhance supportive environments for healthy aging of seniors.

Results of Tests

The data collected from our 200 participants suggests that older adults living at Spanish Cove are above average for most of the test indicators when compared to other seniors. Most resident scored higher than the national average in upper and lower body strength for both women and men in almost every age category. This is likely the result of a variety of exercise classes that focus on functional fitness and strength. Over the course of testing the past four years, many residents improved their upper and lower body strength each year and many maintained their strength.

The six-minute and the two-minute step both test aerobic endurance. We find that these two tests have unique components that directly correlate to many activities of daily living. For instance, there are 24 two-story independent living apartments at Spanish Cove and up to 50 percent of the residents take the stairs on a daily basis, requiring exercise endurance. As Spanish Cove encompasses a large campus, most residents in independent living apartments walk outside to and from the dining hall and to other buildings for programs and exercise classes. Because of this, it is imperative that residents have the aerobic endurance to navigate the campus and stay active and independent. We did note that many residents who performed more steps during the two-minute walk test covered a longer distance during the six-minute walk. Without question, the size and layout of the Spanish Cove campus helps seniors with their aerobic endurance.

Flexibility is a specific area in which the fitness test results indicated Spanish Cove residents need to focus more attention. Overall, lower body flexibility tested higher than upper body in most residents. Another finding was that residents who regularly practiced yoga exercises tested higher overall for flexibility. Reductions in joint mobility normally come with age and can hinder the ability to safely perform needed activities of daily living. Flexibility can be improved by better range of motion in the major muscle-tendon groups through stretching exercises or a class like yoga. Due to difficulties in the upper and lower body flexibility test, Spanish Cove added a gentle chair yoga class to the exercise program this year. We will continue to test for improvement in this area.

Body weight was above average which may be typical of our region of the country and of adults in general. Some seniors were below average while others were just slightly above Body Mass Index (BMI) scores.

The good news is that our data strongly suggests that older adults who choose to live in an environment that focuses on improving and/or maintaining strength and mobility experience a decrease in fall risk and may be shown to have better mobility than many living in their own homes.

Summary

Aging is often associated with declines in physical function that affect vital processes critical to independence, socialization and quality of life. Opportunities for exercise that lead to fitness, efficient functional movement skills and performance of daily tasks are needed to prevent disability among older adults. Exercise programs aimed to equip older adults with neuro motor (balance, coordination and agility), physical (aerobic endurance, muscle strength and flexibility, and functional components of fitness help persons to remain active and independent. Seniors not participating in exercise are encouraged to add one or more exercise routines in order to feel better, live longer and stay independent as long as possible.

References

1. Thomas S, Reading J, Shepherd PJ. Physical Activity Readiness Questionnaire. Canadian J Sport 1992
2. Rikli RE, Jones J. *Senior Fitness Test Manual.* Human Kinetics. 2013. 2nd ed.
3. See 2
4. See 2
5. See 1

Chapter 6
Mental Health

Brain function and mental health inevitably shows some decline as people age, however, there is much that can be done to slow the rate of the decline. The ultimate outcome of brain dysfunction is Alzheimer's disease, a condition that now affects more than five million Americans older than 65, or roughly one in nine. The number of persons affected is expected to triple by 2050. Fortunately, research today indicates there are things we can do—from childhood to older ages—to make the brain less vulnerable to diseases of aging.

The brain is the most plastic and adaptable organ in the body. This plasticity appears to account for our cognitive reserve as well as continued function. While it was once thought that when brain cells die, there is a slow loss of brain activity as the cell numbers decrease but it is now known that brain cells can be regenerated through a process called "neurogenesis". How the brain functions and what influences its actions are under intense study in order to know more about preventing the onset of mental diseases. Genetics plays a role but other lifestyle factors are thought to play an even greater role in overall brain health. The same factors as outlined in Chapter 2 that apply to the aging process also apply to mental health, e.g., exercise, nutrition, social contacts, sleep, control of stress and use of the mind.

The Mind-Body Connection

Researchers know that all life processes are interconnected. For instance, what is good for the heart, the immune system and physical health is also good for the brain. Advances in the treatment of cardiovascular risks, including high blood pressure, diabetes and high cholesterol all lead to better brain health. Vascular problems often lead to heart disease and can also affect brain function by interfering with the supply of oxygen-rich blood that nourishes brain cells.

Mind-body interactions have important implications for the way illness is viewed and treated. A group associated with the Massachusetts General Hospital is looking at the connections made in mind-body medicine. (1) They show that physical health is influenced by thoughts, feelings and behaviors, and conversely, thoughts, feelings and behaviors are influenced by physical symptoms.

Stress, either acute or chronic, can lead to both physical and mental trauma. Hormones are released in a stressful situation, leading to the "fight or flight" syndrome. The digestive system, the nervous system and, in fact, most body systems are affected by stress. Chronic stress can even lead to an increased risk of obesity, insomnia and poor mental function. Inflammatory factors have been shown to be elevated in older persons and may be a risk factor for the development of age-related neurodegenerative disease. (2)

Cognitive Impairment

The Alzheimer's Association defines this mental condition as one resulting from complex interactions among multiple factors: age, genetics, environment, lifestyle and co-existing medical conditions. (3) Some 3.5 million persons in the U.S. have Alzheimer's disease and about a third of these are 85 and older. Added to this statistic are the many others who have lesser forms of dementia that affect both physical and mental health with differing degrees of cognitive impairment.

While aging itself presents a strong risk for the development and progression of cognitive decline, other factors may be of even greater importance. The Alzheimer's Association was asked in 2014 to support evidence of actions associated with the prevention of cognitive decline and dementia. (4) They identified the following:

- Regular physical exercise
- Management of cardiovascular risk factors (diabetes, obesity, high blood pressure)
- A healthy diet
- Lifelong learning
- Cognitive training

The Association lists the following warning signs for the onset of dementia: memory loss that disrupts daily life; challenges in planning and solving problems; difficulty completing familiar tasks at home, work or at leisure; confusion with time or place; trouble understanding visual images and spatial relationships.

Memory loss or memory or memory lapses is a common occurrence as people age. In itself, this does not necessarily mean that a person is developing dementia. Typical activities that most often indicate normal age-related forgetfulness, mild cognitive impairment or dementia are shown in the following chart developed by Johns Hopkins shown on page 38. (5)

Physical Activity

Although the brain represents only two percent of the body mass, it uses about 25 percent of all energy required to operate the body every day. Physical exercise boosts the heart rate, helping to send the needed oxygen, plus blood, hormones and neurotransmitters throughout the body. Exercise has also been shown to increase the mitochondria in cells thus generating and maintaining energy in both muscles and brain (6) Studies further show that getting the heart rate up enhances neurogenesis or the ability to grow new brain cells in adults. There is further indication that habitual moderate exercise rewires the brain and immune system to better cope with physical and mental strain. Especially good at treating depression, exercise seems to mimic chemical effects of anti-depressant medicine. (7)

Distinguishing Normal "Senior Moments" from More Worrisome Memory Lapses		
Occasional memory lapses, such as forgetting why you walked into a room or having difficulty recalling a person's name, become more common as we approach our 50s and 60s. It's comforting to know that this minor forgetfulness is a normal sign of aging, not a sign of dementia. But other types of memory loss, such as for getting appointments or becoming momentarily disoriented in a familiar place, may indicate mild cognitive impairment. In dementia- the most serious form of memory impairment - people often find themselves disoriented In time and place and unable to name common objects or recognize once familiar people. The chart below gives examples of the types of memory problems common in normal age-related forgetfulness, mild cognitive impairment and dementia.		

Normal Age-Related Forgetfulness	Mild Cognitive Impairment	Dementia
Sometimes misplaces keys, eyeglasses or other items.	Frequently forgets people's names and is slow to recall them.	Forgets what an item is used for or puts it in an inappropriate place.
Momentarily forgets an acquaintance's name.	Frequently forgets people's names and is slow to recall them.	May not remember knowing a person.
Occasionally has to "search" for a word.	Has more difficulty using the right words.	Begins to lose language skills. May withdraw from social interaction.
Occasionally forgets to run an errand.	Begins to forget important events and appointments.	Loses sense of time. Doesn't know what day it is
May forget an event from the distant past.	May forget more recent events or newly learned information.	Has serious impairment of short term memory. Has difficulty learning and remembering new information.

When driving, may momentarily forget where to turn; quickly orients self.	May temporarily become lost more often. May have trouble understanding and following a map.	Becomes easily disoriented or lost in familiar places, sometimes for hours.
Jokes about memory loss.	Worries about memory loss. Family and friends notice the lapses.	May have little or no awareness of cognitive problems.

Guide to Understanding Dementia, Johns Hopkins Health, 2009

Using the Brain

Education, both formal and experiential, is beneficial to brain health by building cognitive reserve. The onset of dementia and loss of mental capacity can be significantly delayed by continuing to use the mind. (8) Researchers have also found that other factors later in life can also buy more years of healthy living: purpose, conscientiousness, organization, self-discipline, dependability and a drive to achieve. All these personality traits are thought to offer protection against Alzheimer's. Among physical activities that help the brain are bilingualism, mastering a musical instrument, reading and writing and continuing education activities.

Mental Tests

There are several tests for assessing mental capacity. One often used is the Mini-Mental Examination (MME). (9) This test is often used to detect dementia, which is responsible for most of the loss of cognitive function in older adults. The DETERMINE test is another used for nutritional status that is also associated with symptoms of depression and with lower functional status. (10) This is a ten-question check list that assigns points to specific health practices and gives an interpretation of each item. Other mental tests are used in psychological and clinical diagnoses of mental capacity and indications for treatment.

At Spanish Cove, the MME is administered to all new residents. It is also been used in general fitness/wellness testing sessions for residents. Such an assessment is helpful in determining the type and amount of care provided residents.

Nutrition for Mental Health

"Eat well to keep the mind sharp" is the headline in a recent Health and Nutrition newsletter from Tufts University Nutrition Center. (11) Eating habits throughout life are among the major determinants of successful aging, both physically and mentally. While food intake often declines as age advances, the need for several specific nutrients increases. (See Chapter 8).

The relationship between good dietary habits and optimum mental function is direct and is critically important. Many studies have shown that the DASH diet and the Mediterranean diets are effective in meeting nutritional needs for the older adult and may in fact improve nutritional status. A plan that combines the heart-healthy Mediterranean and DASH plans with even more emphasis on foods and nutrients that boost brain health is the Mediterranean-DASH Intervention for Neurodegenerative Delay (MIND) diet plan. The plan was developed at Rush University and funded by the National Institute on Aging. All three plans emphasize plant-based foods and limited intake of red meat and foods high in saturated fat. Foods providing antioxidants (fruits and vegetables, healthy fats and B vitamins) are emphasized. Ten brain-healthy foods are featured: leafy greens, vegetables, nuts, berries, beans, whole grains, fish, poultry, olive oil, wine.

A complete outline of the MIND diet plan is shown in Appendix B.

Daily Living Activities

A summary of the areas of daily living that are important at all ages for brain health are the following:
1. Following a healthy eating plan
2. Participating in various kinds of physical activity
3. Preventing and/or controlling blood lipids (LDL, HDL, cholesterol)

4. Controlling blood sugar levels
5. Maintaining a healthy weight
6. Staying mentally active
7. Avoiding stress
8. Using alcohol in moderation if at all and not smoking
9. Maintaining social contacts

Summary

Some decline in mental health usually accompanies aging, however, the brain is an adaptable organ that is influenced by a number of lifestyle practices. Cognitive impairment can be delayed and even prevented to an extent by exercise, optimal nutrition and by continual learning and use of the brain. Tests for mental function are often used in assessment of brain health and for making lifestyle changes if indicated.

References

1. Mind-Body Basics. www.massgeneral.org

2. Tan ZS, Seshadri S. Inflammation in the Alzheimer's Disease Cascade. Culprit or Innocent Bystander? Alzheimer's Res. Ther. 2010;2:6.

3. About Alzheimer's disease: Alzheimer's Basics NIA. www.nia.nih.gov/

4. See reference 3

5. Guide to Understanding Dementia. Johns Hopkins Health Alerts. 2009:1.

6. Jahr F. Head Strong. MIND Scientific American Jan/Feb 2017:27-31.

7. How does exercise benefit cognition? MIND. Scientific American Sept/ Oct 2016:72-73.

8. Bennett DA. Banking Against Alzheimer's. Scientific American MIND. July/Aug 2016:3—37.

9. Folstein MF, Folstein SE, McHugh PR. Mini-Mental State: A Practical Method for Grading the Cognitive State of Patients for the Clinician. J Psychiatr 1975;12(3):189-198.

10. Nutrition Screening Initiative. DETERMINE your nutritional health checklist. Washington D. C. Nutrition Screening Initiative 1991. www. aafp.org

11. Eat well to keep the mind sharp. Tufts U. Health and Nutrition Newsletter. 2017;34(12):1,3

Chapter 7
Mindful Eating

Our food choices are strongly influenced by the habits we form throughout life. Food preferences based on taste, availability and cost along with knowledge about healthful food choices are all factors. Health-related influences such as food allergies and the need for special diets will also affect choices. Nestle (1), in her book *What to Eat* makes a strong point about how food marketing and food processing practices have a large and perhaps outsized impact on what people choose to eat. Realizing that there are many things that influence our food choices, giving thought to the impact of those choices is worthwhile and likely to benefit our health over time.

Mindful eating refers to simply being aware of one's needs, food choices, amount eaten and the environmental circumstances such as home, restaurant or other institution, all of which can affect food behavior. Such awareness can help control overeating, making poor food choices and, eventually, lead to overall good health. (2) Mindful eating is critical during fast-growing periods of life as in childhood and teenage years because growth and development is dependent on food choices. During the adult years, the ground work is being laid for continued health or for slowly developing chronic conditions that may play a large role in their effect on body systems later in life. In the older adult, emphasis on eating choices is of continued importance in helping maintain strength and fitness and for resisting disease.

As a practice, eating thoughtfully can be characterized in several ways. First, food choices not only affect health but also affect the environment. Through awareness and consideration of scientific recommendations on nutrition, a person can adopt dietary patterns that are lower in red and processed meats and higher in plant foods, thus leading to lower incidences of chronic diseases. Concern for how food is produced and its effect on animal welfare and workers in the agriculture industry may follow.

Understanding *why* we eat what we do means having knowledge about nutrition, the influence of advertising and food marketers as well as foods available on the market. *How much* to eat is a further part of making food choices based on physiological need and also about managing emotions that drive eating. Whether to "eat to live" or "live to eat" is a seemingly simple way of characterizing the food choices one makes and the amounts. It can also demonstrate mindfulness toward the amount of food eaten. *How to eat* involves appreciation for the taste, smell, sight, sound and texture of food eaten in non-distracting surroundings. Eating then becomes enjoyable and raises awareness of the human and natural resources that brought it to us.

A conceptual model illustrating the use of mindful eating for health promotion and sustainability is shown in Figure 1. Developing an awareness of relationships between food and our body as well as our environment helps maintain our health and the health of the larger community.

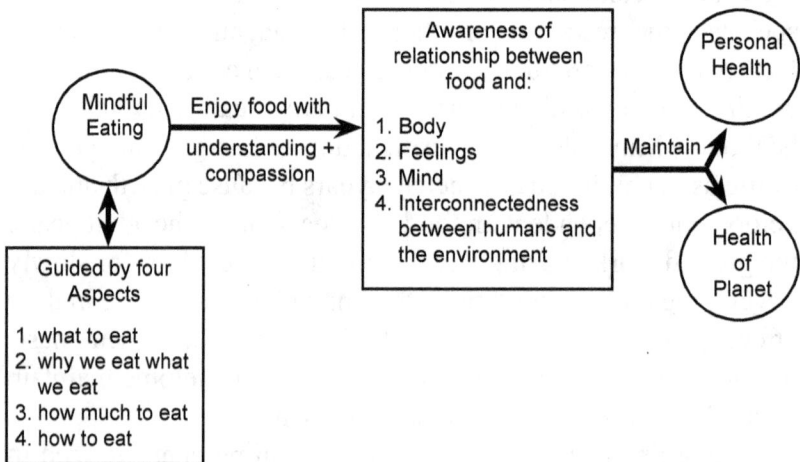

Figure 1. Model for Mindful Eating
Source: Reference 2

Food Choices

There are several nutritionally sound plans that have been shown to promote good health and help stave off the onset of chronic disease. Lichtenstein (3), a vice-chair of the Dietary Guidelines committee and Tufts University professor, says that dietary patterns are more important than specific foods when it comes to making food choices. A healthy dietary pattern is adaptable to cultural and ethnic concerns and can and should taste and look good. Such plans are higher in vegetables, fruit, whole grain, low or nonfat dairy, seafood, legumes and nuts and moderate in alcohol, lower in red and processed meat and low in sugar-sweetened foods and drinks. The simplest eating plan is illustrated in MyPlate (shown below). Developed by the U.S. Department of Agriculture, the plan shows that at least half the intake should come from fruits and vegetables with lesser amounts from grains, meats and dairy products. Directions for using MyPlate translated into meals can be found at www.usda.cnnp.gov.

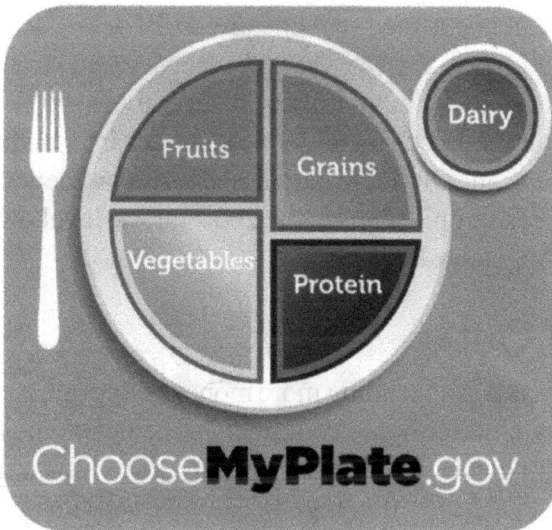

DASH DIET. A highly recommended eating plan, the "Dietary Approach to Stop Hypertension" (DASH) was developed by the National Heart, Lung, and Blood division of the National

Institutes of Health. The plan was a part of a national effort to drive down the prevalence of high blood pressure among the population. Not only has the diet plan helped do this very effectively but has also been shown to be effective in weight loss, decreased cholesterol levels and improvement of insulin sensitivity. The emphasis in the plan is on fruits and vegetables, decreased sodium, vegetable rather than animal fats and less red meat. The diet outline is shown in Appendix C.

MEDITERRANEAN DIET. The Mediterranean diet plan is one adapted from that area of the world that has also been shown to promote good nutritional health. The Mayo Clinic describes the diet as a "heart-healthy" plan based on typical foods and recipes of Mediterranean-style cooking. (4) It has been associated with a reduced incidence of cancer, Parkinson's disease and Alzheimer's disease. Evidence of brain benefits from following a Mediterranean staple diet is shown in a large-scale study called PREDIMED. The findings from the study show that people who closely follow this eating plan are more likely to maintain their memory and thinking skills over time. (5, 6).

The plan is outlined in Appendix D.

USDA DIET PLANS. The U.S. Department of Agriculture publishes outlines of eating plans at several calorie levels. They are based on the Dietary Guidelines and are intended to help in meal planning and food selection based on recommended nutrient intakes. Three sample plans at the 2000 calorie level of intake are shown in Appendix E.

Eating Out

Americans are spending more money eating out at restaurants than buying food for home cooking.(7) The potential for making less-healthy choices when eating out is a reality. Restaurant meals, for the most part, are often high in calories, sodium and sugar. In regard to calorie counting, studies have shown that most people underestimate the calorie content of restaurant meals or identify the entrée as highest in calories. This will become easier as restaurants meeting certain size requirements are now requested to post this information for their menus.

Another problem is in estimating serving sizes, especially since many restaurants tend to serve very large portions. Some examples of how to translate portion sizes using familiar objects are shown in the sidebar. (8) Unfamiliarity with menu terms may also limit good choices.

Several suggestions for helping make good choices when eating out are the following:

- Develop a healthy mindset that prevents looking at every meal out as an occasion to throw caution to the wind.
- Choose restaurants that make it easier to eat healthfully and be aware that many fast food restaurants offer the least healthy options.
- Think about the day's choices before ordering, Skipping breakfast or lunch to save up can lead to the temptation to order too much.
- Practice portion control. Stay away from terms like "jumbo", "grande", "supreme" etc.
- If possible, ask for half, lunch or appetizer portions. Choose from a la carte items and/or side offerings, mixing and matching to make a meal. Split or share or take home part of the food.
- Practice menu creativity, i.e., start with a salad or soup, then the appetizer.
- Ask for foods as you want them, such as a specific cooking method, leaving out an ingredient or a substitution.
- Recognize when internal cues say the body has had enough.

Dietary Supplements

Multivitamin-Minerals

The question as to whether older persons should, as a precautionary measure, take multivitamin and mineral supplements should be determined by whether there is an underlying condition that would be benefitted from a nutritional standpoint. Most nutrition authorities agree that they are needed in a deficiency such as chronic illness, malnutrition or poor eating habits due to lack of appetite. Other indicators for possible supplement need are antioxidants for macular degeneration, B-12 in a lack of stomach acid, iron for postmenopausal women, and vitamin D

TAKE CHARGE!

It's most accurate to weigh or measure food portions, but that's not always practical. Eyeballing portions by comparing them to everyday objects can help.

Lean meat; skinless chicken breast Portion: 3 oz cooked Average calories: 135 Size of: deck of cards	
Main-dish casserole Portion: 1 cup Average calories: 310 Size of: baseball	
Starchy vegetables (corn, potatoes, peas) Portion: 1/2 cup Average calories: 80 Size of: cupcake wrapper	
Spaghetti Portion: 2 oz dry Average calories: 200 Size of: nickel (diameter of bundle)	
Dried fruit Portion: 1/4 cup Average calories: 120 Size of: lrage egg	
Nuts Portion: 1 oz Average calories: 170 Size of: lsmall shot glass	
Hard cheese Portion: 1 oz Average calories: 100 Size of: domino	
Peanut butter Portion: 2 tablespoons Average calories: 190 Size of: golf ball	

for osteoporotic bones. For the healthy older person, the best practice is to eat a wide variety of foods, thereby gaining the needed nutrients in the right amount.

Studies on multivitamin-mineral intake for heart health have shown little or no effect although if taken for 20 years or more, there may be some positive effect in men. A large-scale Women's Health Study also showed no benefit for preventing cardiovascular events including heart attacks, strokes and death. (9)

Persons who do take vitamin-mineral supplements need to be aware of the safe upper limit for each as determined by the Food and Nutrition Board of the National Academy of Sciences who have established a safe upper limit on most vitamins and minerals. The risk of adverse effects including specific toxicities can occur if intakes exceed established levels. (10)

Protein Supplements

Older adults tend to lose body protein with changes in body composition. Added to such loss, there is often a decrease in appetite along with functional and social limitations among many. (11) When such loss occurs, extra protein, especially animal protein, is needed to spare muscle loss. Protein supplements that provide protein, carbohydrate and other added nutrients are also a way of increasing intake. Several high protein products are on the market that can be helpful, especially when whole foods are not taken due to lack of appetite or difficulty in chewing or swallowing.

Dietary Supplements

The National Center for Complementary and Alternative Medicine (NCCAM) of the National Institutes of Health says Americans spend billions of dollars each year on dietary supplements. They are sold over-the-counter without a prescription and include amino acids, herbs, botanicals and enzymes. Dietary supplements are substances that come in the form of pills, capsules, powders, gel tabs and extracts. The Food and Drug Administration does not monitor them in the same way as prescription medicines and is not allowed to restrict their sale or use due to the 1994 Dietary Supplement and Health Education Act (DSHEA). By this act, the manufacturers, not the Food and Drug Administration certify that their product is safe and does what it promises. (12) However, many dietary supplements are not fully tested for either safety or efficacy and the consumer has no way of knowing this. Some supplements can interact with medicines, leading to life-threatening situations. These are most often herbals such as ginseng, gingko biloba, St. John's wort, or echinacea.

Probiotics are another type of supplement that are used to maintain the body's balance of intestinal microorganisms. They come in powders, liquids or pills made up of live bacteria. Fermented foods and yogurt also provide the bacteria. As with other supplements, probiotics arc not regulated by the Food and Drug Administration and their value has not been fully proven. (14)

Fish oil, containing omega-3's, has been shown to protect against heart disease. Studies pooled and analyzed from 76 countries show that higher levels of omega-3 oils are associated with a lower risk of dying from heart attacks. While studies have shown conflicting results regarding supplements in general, all agree that omega-3 oils are beneficial and that fish consumption is probably the best way to obtain these oils. Some seeds and nuts are also good sources. The same benefit from fish holds for brain health and mental decline. Eating fish appears to be of more value than taking supplements. (15)

Summary

Eating mindfully is a way of making good food choices for good nutrition, good health and personal satisfaction. Several eating patterns are recommended that meet nutritional requirements and can help control weight and prevent the early onset of chronic disease among older adults. Food supplements may be useful adjuncts to foods depending on the type, the reason for taking them and an understanding of both beneficial and harmful effects.

References

1. Nestle M. "What to Eat". North Point, Publisher. New York. N.Y. 2006

2. Fung TT, Long MW, Hung P, Cheung LWV. An Expanded Model for Mindful Eating for Health Promotion and Sustainability: Issues and Challenges for Dietetics Practice. J Acad Nutr Diet 2016;116(7):1081-1086.

3. Lichtenstein A. 5 Things the Nutrition Experts want you to Know. Tufts U. Health and Nutrition Newsletter 2015;33(3):1.

4. www.mayoclinic.org/healthy_lifestyle/nutrition

5. Mediterranean Diet: Good for your Heart and Mind. Harvard Heart Newsletter. 2015;25(12):1,7.

6. New Evidence of Brain Benefits from following a Mediterranean Diet. Tufts U. Health and Nutrition Newsletter 2015;33(6):1,3.

7. Smart Strategies for Eating Out. Tufts U. Health and Nutrition Newsletter. 2015;9:1,4.

8. Mastering Portion Control. Tufts U. Health and Nutrition Newsletter. 2017;34(1):4-5.

9. Benefits of Multivitamins for Heart Health Needs. Tufts U. Health and Nutrition Newsletter. 2017;34(12):6.

10. No Heart Benefit Seen for Women taking Multivitamins. Tufts U. Health and Nutrition Newsletter 2015;32(1):3.

11. Bernstein M., Munoz N. "Nutrition for the Older Adult." 2nd ed. Jones and Bartlett, Burlington, MA. 2016.

12. Supplements: A Complete Guide to Safety. Consumer Reports. 2016:20-27.

13. Blood Levels of Omega-3s from fish, plants linked to low fatal heart attacks. Tufts U. Health and Nutrition Newsletter 2016;34(8)3.

14. Fish oil Supplements fail to Prevent Mental Decline. Tufts U. Health and Nutrition Newsletter 2015;32(10):7.

15. Schardt D. Are Probiotics Worth Taking? Nutrition Action Newsletter, 2015;Jan-Feb:9-11.

Chapter 8
Nutritional Health

As persons age, their body metabolism slows. There is a tendency to use less energy in physical activity along with loss of muscle tissue, all of which leads to the need for fewer calories. But as calories drop with age, there remains a need for all other nutrients at approximately the same level for the body to work at peak efficiency. Obtaining the same number of nutrients but with fewer calories can be a problem especially if overall food intake is decreased. By some estimates, as many as 25 percent of Americans in their 60's and older have some degree of malnutrition. This does not mean the evidence of deficiency disease but may mean subclinical deficiencies that have a harmful effect on body performance.

The adequacy of nutrient intake is determined by referring to the Dietary Reference Intakes (DRI). The DRI are values determined by the Food and Nutrition Board of the National Academy of Sciences based on research and statistical applications. (1) They indicate the relationship between nutrient intakes and dietary adequacy as well as the prevention of chronic diseases in healthy populations. The DRI include four reference values which apply to known amounts of nutrients. The values and their definition are the following:

- Estimated Average Requirement (EAR). The level estimated to meet the requirements of half of the healthy individuals in a particular life stage and gender group.
- Recommended Dietary Allowance (RDA). The average daily dietary nutrient intake that meets the nutrient requirements of 97-98 percent of healthy individuals in a particular life stage and gender group.

- Adequate Intake (AI). Estimates of nutrient intake by a group of apparently healthy people assumed to be adequate; used when an RDA cannot be determined.
- Upper Level (UL). The tolerable upper limit is the highest average daily intake that is likely to pose no risk of adverse health effects to almost all individuals in the general population. The DRI's for the 70 plus age male and female are shown in Appendix H.

Relationship of Nutrients to Overall Health

Health and well-being are influenced by numerous inter-related factors over a lifetime. Nutrition is a major determinant in successful aging. It has been shown that some 85 percent of non-institutionalized older adults have one or more chronic health conditions that could be improved with good or better nutrition and up to half may have clinical evidence of malnutrition. (2). Many of these illnesses limit activity along with functional independence and quality of life.

Consumption of a poor-quality diet can result in inadequate intakes of energy and essential nutrients, resulting in malnutrition and worsening health status. Malnourished older adults are more prone to infections and diseases, their injuries take longer to heal, surgery is riskier and hospital stays are longer and more expensive.

Nutrients play important roles in body metabolism and maintenance. They act as co-factors in enzyme reactions, provide energy, function in the immune system, carry oxygen to cells, build bones and muscle, allow the brain to function and more. The effect of insufficient or excessive amounts of nutrients or the development of health-related diseases is not fully known, however research has provided a great deal of information as to the causal relationship. For instance, it is now known that the development of dementia, especially Alzheimer's disease, is due partly to genetics but perhaps even more importantly, to lifestyle factors throughout life. Along with exercise, sleep, non-smoking, control of stress and social contacts, nutrition is a leading factor. So many reactions and functions in body metabolism are dependent on adequate sources of specific nutrients that their intake cannot be over-emphasized.

The way that a poor diet deficient in nutrients affects the older adult is shown in Figure 1.

Nutrition and Food Selection

The practice of good nutrition begins with food selection from choices offered or from food purchased. Buying decisions are aided by information provided about foods and their contents. For instance, nutrition labels on foods yield a great deal of information about particular nutrients in the product with the amounts and also the percentage of daily need provided by each nutrient. The Nutrient Labeling Education Act (NLEA) 0f 1990 authorized the Food and Drug Administration (FDA) to provide

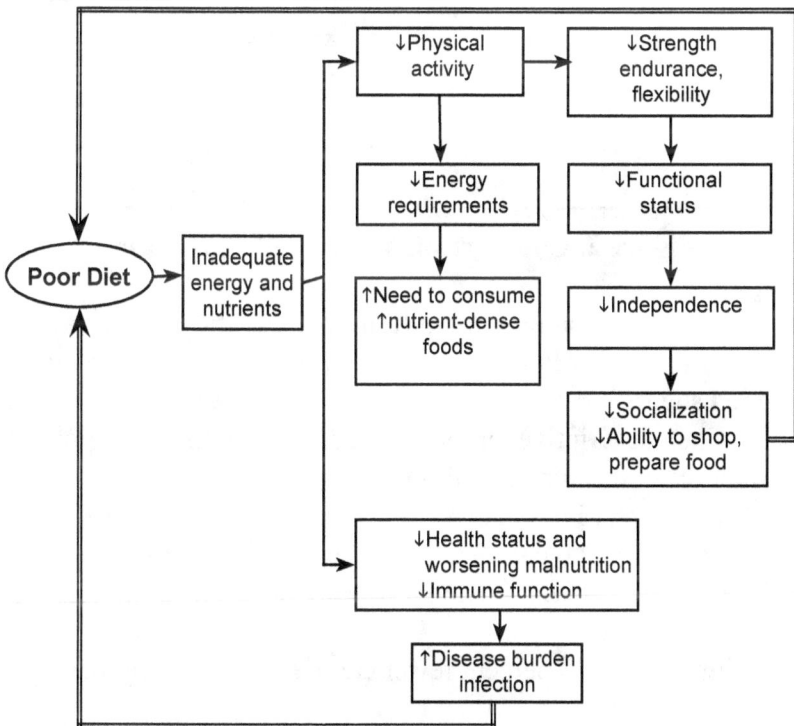

Figure 1. Poor Diet Affects the Older Adult
Source: Bernstein M, Munson H. Nutrition for the Older Adult. Jones and Bartlett, Burlington, MA 2016.

nutrition labeling on foods regulated by the FDA and also defined
health claims that could be made on products. The label is being
updated and a new format will be in effect in 2020. A depiction
of both the present and the new format is shown in Figure 2.

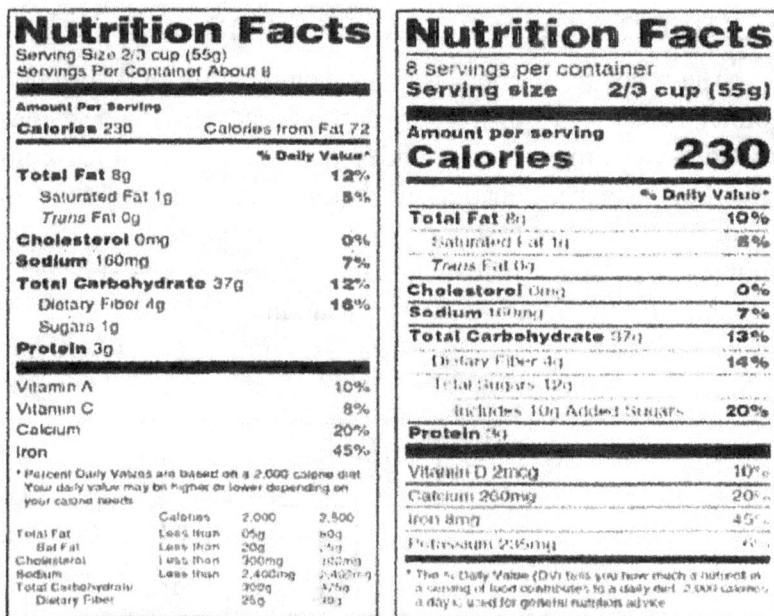

Figure 2. Comparison of Old and New Label

The main changes include more realistic serving sizes,
calories appear in large print and the addition of the category
"added sugars".

When descriptive terms are used, regulations also apply as
to their exact meaning as follows:
- Calorie-free. Less than 5 calories per serving.
- Low calorie. 40 calories or less per serving.
- Reduced calorie. 25 percent fewer calories than the original
  food item.
- Light or lite. 33 percent fewer calories than the original food
  item.
- Reduced fat. 25 percent less fat per serving than the original
  item.
- Low fat. Three grams of fat or less per serving.

- Fat free. Less than 0.5 grams of fat per serving.
- Reduced sodium. At least 25 percent less than in the original item.
- Salt or sodium free. Less than 5 mg of sodium per serving.
- Low sodium. 140 mg or less per serving.
- Light in sodium or lightly salted. At least 50 percent less than the regular food.

Definitions of descriptive terms are the following:

"Excellent source of"—20 percent or higher of the Daily Value of nutrient per serving.

"Good source"—10-19 percent of the Daily Value of nutrient per serving.

"Enriched with"—Vitamins or minerals removed during processing but added back.

"Fortified with"—Vitamins or minerals not naturally in foods so is being added.

Nutrient--Disease Claims

Several health claims have been approved and may be used in describing the relationship between certain nutrients and disease. Those currently approved that may be used are the following:

Disease	Beneficial Nutrients	Adverse-effect Nutrients
Cancer	Fiber-containing grains, fruits, vegetables	Dietary lipids
Coronary heart disease	Fruits, vegetables, soy protein, soluble fiber grains, stanols, sterols	Saturated fat, cholesterol
Neural tube defects	Folic acid	
Osteoporosis	Calcium, Vitamin D	
Hypertension	Sodium	

Nutrition Screening and Assessment

Nutrition screening helps identify individuals who are at nutritional risk or who are malnourished. Patterns of dietary intake reflect a person's habitual consumption of food and beverages and can help determine nutritional risk. Several nutrition screening instruments have been developed for use with older adults. Once a screening procedure has shown needed improvement in a person's nutritional status, further assessment is done in order to initiate corrective action as needed.

Two of the most widely used screening instruments are the *Nutrition Screening Initiative (NSI)* and the *Mini Nutritional Assessment (MNA)*. (3,4) The NSI includes a self-assessment questionnaire of ten questions that are associated with nutritional health in older adults. Low scores indicate a low risk of poor nutritional status. The ten questions and scores are the following:

1. I have an illness or condition that made me change the kind/amount of food I eat. 2
2. I eat fewer than 2 meals a day. 3
3. I eat few fruits or vegetables or milk products. 2
4. I have 3 or more drinks of beer, liquor, or wine almost every day. 2
5. I have tooth or mouth problems that make it hard to eat. 2
6. I don't always have enough money to buy the food I need. 4
7. I eat alone most of the time. 1
8. I take 3 or more different prescribed or over-the –counter drugs a day. 1
9. Without wanting to, I have lost or gained 10 pounds in the last 6 months. 2
10. I am not always physically able to shop, cook, and/or feed myself. 2

    (Score of 0-2 is good; 3-5 means moderate nutritional risk; 6 or more means high nutritional risk.)

A nutrition checklist is based on warning signs described below, the first letter in each forming the word DETERMINE.

* **Disease.** Any disease, illness or chronic condition that makes It hard to eat puts nutritional health at risk. Sadness or depression can cause big changes in appetite, digestion, energy level, weight and well-being.
* **Eating poorly.** Eating too little or too much both lead to poor health. Eating the same thing day after day or not eating, fruits,

vegetables and dairy products cause poor nutritional health.

- **Tooth loss/mouth pain.** A healthy mouth, teeth and gums are needed to eat well.
- **Economic hardship.** As many as 40 percent of older Americans have low incomes. Having or spending less for food makes it hard to get the foods needed for health.
- **Reduced social contact.** One-third of older people live alone. Being with people daily has a positive effect on morale, well-being and eating.
- **Multiple medicines.** The more medicines taken, the greater chance for side effects such as change in taste, constipation, weakness, drowsiness, diarrhea, nausea, and others. Even vitamins and minerals taken in large amounts can cause harm.
- **Involuntary weight gain or loss.** Losing or gaining a lot of weight when not trying is a warning sign that increases the chance of poor health.
- **Needs assistance in self-care.** Trouble walking, shopping and cooking food are health risks.
- **Elder years above age 80.** As age increases, the risk of frailty and health problems increase.

A person who has been identified to be at nutritional risk may then undergo a more complete assessment that includes anthropometric, biochemical, clinical and dietary evaluation. The components of each of the measurements are as follows:

Anthropometric: weight, height, BMI, skinfolds, body composition.

Biochemical: protein status, cholesterol level, vitamin and mineral status.

Clinical: medical history, signs and symptoms, cognitive and physical function, oral health, medication use.

Dietary: food and beverage intake, food security, supplement use, food preferences, cultural practices.

The Mini Nutritional Assessment is composed of two sections: six questions for screening and further questions with anthropometric measures if the risk of malnutrition is shown. The six questions address weight loss, acute illness, mobility, dementia or depression and appetite and intake changes. A score is given showing sign of or risk of malnutrition. The MNA has been validated and shown to be a reliable measure of nutritional health. The screening and assessment questions may be found at www.mna_elderly.com.

Sarcopenia Risk Assessment. A recent report in the Journal of Nutrition describes research for the risk of sarcopenia among 274 community-dwelling older persons. (5) A questionnaire, composed of seven questions, described as related to the risk of sarcopenia, was used. The questions covered age, protein and dairy consumption, number of meals per day, physical activity level, number of hospitalizations and weight loss in the past year. The conclusion of the study was that the questions were predictive of sarcopenia and could be used as a prescreening instrument.

Summary

Nutritional health, along with physical and mental health, is a significant factor in how people age and how long they live. It is one of the leading indicators along with exercise and other lifestyle practices that define a person's quality of life during the later years. Learning to check nutrient content of foods and the relationships between various nutrients and diseases is important in food selection for nutrient content. Finally, screening for nutritional status helps identify risks for maintaining a heathy lifestyle as well as physical fitness.

References

1. Dietary Reference Intakes. National Academies Press. Institute of Medicine. Washington D.C. 2006.

2. Chernoff R. "Geriatric Nutrition: The Health Professionals Handbook" Jones and Bartlett, Sudbury, MA 2006:6-9.

3. Nutrition Screening Initiative. Report of Nutrition Screening I: Toward a Common View. Washington D.C. 1991.

4. Skates JJ, Anthony P. The Mini Nutritional Assessment—An Integral Part of Geriatric Assessment. Nutr Today 2009;44(1):21-28.

5. Rossi AP, Micciolo R, Rubole S, et al. Assessing the Risk of Sarcopenia in the Elderly: The Mini Sarcopenia Risk Assessment (MSRA) Questionnaire. J Nutr Health Aging. 2017. Doi.10.1007/s12603-017-0-21-4.

Chapter 9
Healthy Weight—Too Much and Too Little

Many people tend to add weight beginning at about middle age. There are several factors that may be involved: hormones, slowdown of metabolism, less exercise, decreased muscle mass or other lifestyle practices. Data from the Centers for Disease Control shows that 38.5 percent of men and 31.2 percent of women age 65 to 74 years exercise regularly, whereas only 23 percent of men and 14 percent age 75 and older participate in regular exercise thus predisposing them toward weight gain. (1) Changes in body composition also occur as noted in an earlier chapter which may affect weight. Loss of lean muscle mass accelerates after about age 60 along with an increase in fat mass. The reduction in lean body mass accompanied by a decrease in strength is termed sarcopenia.

Changes in the endocrine system can be contributing factor in weight change in the older adult. Hypothyroidism is said to increase fivefold in persons 80 years of age and older, causing a slowdown in body metabolism. The reduction of estrogen in women and testosterone in men as well as a gradual decrease in growth hormone are also thought to be involved. (2) Increased insulin resistance in the aging adult can also promote fat deposition. Even oxidative stress that increases with age is a factor in almost all chronic diseases, including obesity. (3)

Adverse Effects of Obesity

Many chronic diseases are closely linked to obesity including diabetes, high blood pressure and blood lipid abnormalities. Other conditions are joint pain, sleep apnea and respiratory problems. Even some cancers are linked to obesity such as breast, colon, gallbladder and uterine in women and prostate cancer is obese men. (4) Metabolic abnormalities also increase with obesity as in the metabolic syndrome that includes hypertension, elevated blood glucose, central adiposity and abnormal cholesterol levels. (5) Plasma glucose increases each decade after age 30 with a higher prevalence of diabetes in the older adult. Increases in weight may be a leading factor in the development of diabetes and insulin resistance.

Even given the many adverse effects of obesity on health, epidemiologic evidence shows that mild overweight may actually have a protective effect against mortality in the older adult. What is lacking is guidance toward how much weight can be considered optimal and the point at which it becomes detrimental. On an individual basis, evaluating the benefits of weight loss against the possible risks in the older adult appears to be the best approach.

Managing Weight

Due to the loss of height and body composition changes with aging, current weight standards (Body Mass Index) for the older adult may not be appropriate in the same way as for younger adults. Researchers suggest that weight maintenance, eating a healthy diet and participating in physical fitness activities all help maintain functional status and strength. These may be the most desirable actions rather than weight loss per se.

The Body Mass Index (BMI) is, at present, the most reliable reference available on a population-wide basis for determining desirable weight ranges. The BMI chart is included in Appendix F as a general reference guide. Other ways of determining healthy weight such as the waist-to-hip measurement, skin caliper measurements or shape (apple or pear) are usually not as effective in the older adult, again due to body changes.

For adults over age 70, the Dietary Reference Intakes (DRI) for men and women are shown in Appendix G. As indicated earlier, the amount of physical exercise affects the total calorie need. The determination of the actual number of calories needed to effect weight loss can be based on the desired rate of loss. Simply put, one pound of fat equals 3500 calories. To lose 1 to 2 pounds a week, it is necessary to decrease calorie intake by 500-1000 a day.

There is no one standard plan for weight reduction. Several plans have been developed, researched extensively and proven to be successful. Two leading ones are the Dietary Approaches to Stop Hypertension (DASH) and the Mediterranean plan. The DASH plan (see Appendix C) was developed to reduce hypertension in persons with moderate to high blood pressure. It encourages consumption of fruits, vegetables, whole grains, nuts, legumes, seed, low-fat dairy products and lean meats. It limits consumption of sodium, caffeinated and alcoholic drinks. Weight loss occurs when the diet is followed. (6)

The Mediterranean diet reflects the usual eating pattern of the European countries in an earlier time. (Appendix D) It is focused on fruits, vegetables, grains, nuts, olive oil as the fat source, dairy products, fish and poultry in low to moderate amounts with very little red meat. Only minimally processed foods are used and calories need to be restricted. Persons following this plan can lose weight and can also improve cardiovascular and brain health. (7, 8)

The U.S. Department of Agriculture also publishes eating plans at a range of calorie levels which can also be used as a guide to food selection for weight loss. The plans are shown in Appendix E.

A theory for weight reduction tentatively discussed in the 2015 Dietary Guidelines and strongly proposed by Taubes (9) is one that drastically reduces all carbohydrates on the basis that insulin production, when overtaxed as in obesity, leads to hyperinsulinism and to the metabolic syndrome. This, in turn, leads to other chronic diseases. The sample diet plans feature meat and very low- carbohydrate containing vegetables but little else. The plan resembles earlier diet regimes such as the Atkins diet and others that feature meats and fats in almost any amount but which have not been universally popular or proven superior to plans more closely resembling normal ways of eating.

When Weight Gain Is Needed

Older adults who are underweight may or may not actually be malnourished but are considered to be at risk for malnutrition. A low BMI status, decreased muscle mass and increased fat mass may be indications for poor nutritional status. A diminished appetite, poor-fitting dentures or swallowing difficulties can lead to weight loss. Depression can also be a factor in unplanned weight loss.

Excessive weight loss may point to undiagnosed disease and leave a person prone to infection and a decrease in independence. It may also mean instability when muscle loss occurs with the risk of falls and broken bones.

Identifying the cause of unwanted weight loss is a medical concern. Cancer is a common reason, accounting for some 19 to 36 percent of cases of unintentional weight loss in older adult. Other chronic diseases may also be involved such as rheumatoid arthritis, Parkinson's disease, digestive disease, alcohol-related disease, and dementia. (10) Congestive heart disease and chronic obstruction pulmonary disease mean that more energy is being used to sustain function of the heart and lungs. Thyroid disease may also increase energy usage.

Another simple reason is poor appetite from decreased smell and taste in addition to decreased thirst. Some prescription medicines can also alter smell and taste or lead to other side effects that dampen appetite. Once the underlying cause of unwanted weight loss is determined, a treatment plan that may combine physical activity and a nutritious diet should be planned on an individual basis. This can include smaller meals at regularly scheduled times, adding spices to foods, high protein and high carbohydrate foods and attention to individual likes and dislikes. Liquid high protein supplements can be used as a snack between meals but not as a meal replacement.

Summary

Maintaining a healthy and stable weight is important for healthy aging. Researchers suggest that weight parameters for older adults do not necessarily follow the same guidelines as for younger adults, given the physical and lifestyle changes that older adults usually experience. Obesity is now considered a national crisis and is a growing concern in many older populations. Many chronic diseases are closely linked to obesity, leading to a poor quality of life and shortened lifespan. Weight loss, on the other hand, may signify chronic disease onset, physical instability and greater risk of infection due to a depressed immune system.

References

1. Administration on Aging. Get Moving! Exercise can Enhance and Extend Your Life. U.S. Department of Health and Human Services. Washington, D.C.

2. Apostalopoulow M et al. Review: Age, Weight and Obesity. Maturitos. 2012;71:115-119.

3. Chandler-Laney PC, Phodke RP, Granger WM et al. Age-related Changes in Insulin Sensitivity and B-cell Activity among European-American and African-American Women. Obesity 2011;19(3):528-535.

4. The Body Weight and Cancer Connection. Health After 50 Newsletter. 2017;28(1):1-2.

5. Expanding Waistlines and Metabolic Syndrome: Researchers warn you of new "Silent Killer". www.Sciencedaily.com/releases2017.

6. Position of the Academy of Nutrition and Dietetics: Interventions for the Treatment of Overweight and Obesity in Adults. J Acad Nutr Diet 2016;116(1):129-147.

7. New Evidence of Brain Benefits from Following a Mediterranean Diet. Tufts U. Health and Nutrition Newsletter. 2015;32(6):1-3.

8. Mediterranean Diet: Good for Your Mind and Your Heart. Harvard Health Letter. 2015;25(12):1,7.

9. Taubes G. "Why we Get Fat and What to do About It. " Anchor Books, Pub. New York, N.Y. 2010.

10. Fighting Unwanted Weight Loss. Tufts U. Health and Nutrition Newsletter. 2017;35(1):6.

Chapter 10

Dietary Guidelines and Health Goals for The U.S.

The *Dietary Guidelines for Americans* were first developed jointly by the U.S. Department of Agriculture and the Department of Health and Human Services in 1980. They were in response to growing concerns and expanded research showing relationships between chronic diseases and nutrition. They were preceded by and replaced the *Dietary Goals* which were developed in 1976 by a Senate committee. Since the initial document was published, the guidelines have been updated and released every five years-- the latest in 2015. The guidelines represent science-based food and nutrition advice for healthy Americans age 2 and older to promote health and prevent chronic diseases. They are also used as a policy guide and as a basis for community education.

Prior to 1980, dietary advice was in the form of eating plans such as the Basic Four and Basic Seven food groups, but with increased research and interest in the relationships between nutrients, dietary excesses and diseases, the guidelines helped set a new direction. An earlier report, the *Surgeon General's Report on Health Promotion and Disease Prevention* reflected a need to further study the relationships between dietary practices and health outcomes. The present eating plan that reflects the guidelines is MyPlate.

The guidelines have grown over the years. From a one-page trifold outlining seven recommendations in 1980, the 2015 guidelines include well over 200 pages of back-up research and discussion supporting the recommendations. The current guidelines provide five major recommendations with multiple areas under each.

The first set of recommendations were more than dietary advice—they included advice for healthy living and nutrients to be avoided in excessive amounts. They were not specific in regard to amounts, instead using phrases such as "too much ", "do in moderation" etc. In this regard, they were general directions. The seven guidelines were the following:

- Eat a variety of foods
- Maintain ideal weight
- Avoid too much fat, saturated fat and cholesterol
- Eat foods with adequate starch and fiber
- Avoid too much sugar
- Avoid too much sodium
- If alcohol is used, do so in moderation

The next several editions were remarkably similar to the first set but included more description. In 2000, 10 recommendations were made which were later condensed. In 2015, five general groups with multiple recommendations with further explanation and background information were issued. The 2015-2020 Guidelines are the following:

1, Follow a healthy eating pattern across the lifespan.

- Account for all food and beverages at the appropriate calorie level.
- Include fruits, vegetables, grains, fat-free or low-fat dairy, proteins.
- Limit saturated and trans fats, added sugars, sodium, alcohol
- Support nutritional adequacy
- Reduce risk of chronic disease
- Include exercise as part of a healthy lifestyle
- Maintain a healthy body weight

2. Focus on variety, nutrient density and amount.
- Variety: for color, flavor, satisfaction, nutrient content
- Nutrient density: to avoid an imbalance of calories and nutrients
- Amount: for meeting recommended nutrient/calorie levels

3. Limit calories from added sugars, saturated fat, reduce sodium
- Added sugars at 10% or less of total calories
- Saturated fat at 10% or less of total calories
- Sodium. 2300 mg per day (1 teaspoon)
- Alcohol. 1 drink per day for women and 2 for men

4. Shift to healthier food and beverage choices.
Studies show that about 75% of the population have low intakes of vegetables, fruits and dairy. More than 50% meet or exceed total grain and protein need but not necessarily, whole grain and healthier types of protein.

5. Support healthy eating patterns for all.
Social and cultural norms that are based on societal values influence eating patterns. Examples are certain types of food, attitudes about body weight and the value placed on physical activity. Food should be accessible for all and food insecurity overcome. An emphasis is placed on support of community programs that provide food and nutrition education such as the Senior Nutrition program offering a meal a day for all seniors.

Throughout all discussions of nutritional health, physical exercise is emphasized as one of the most critical factors in ongoing health. The Dietary Guidelines recommend the following: " in addition to consuming a healthy eating pattern, physical activity is one of the most important things individuals can do to improve their health". Strong evidence shows that regular physical activity helps maintain a healthy weight or reach a healthy weight. Regular exercise also lowers the risk of early death, coronary heart disease, stroke, high blood pressure, poor blood lipid profile, Type 2 diabetes, breast and colon cancer and metabolic syndrome. It can also reduce depression and prevent falls.

The key changes that were made in the 2015-2020 Guidelines were based on the continuing flow of new information available to the drafting committee. For instance, our state of knowledge has advanced regarding caffeine, sugar, sodium, cholesterol, saturated and trans-fats. More detail on eating patterns and nutrients was possible and a shift was made from recommending single foods and/or nutrients to eating patterns.

How Are We Doing?

The chronic diseases responsible for the greatest number of deaths in the U.S. continue to be ones linked to poor diets and little physical exercise. They include heart disease, diabetes and cancer. Further, some two-thirds of Americans are now overweight or obese thus predisposing them to the onset of chronic disease.

The Healthy Eating Index (HEI), a measure developed by the U.S. Department of Agriculture, is calculated from intake studies designed to show diet quality in terms of conformance to the Dietary Guidelines. (1) Using a measure of 100, the scores for older adults over the age of 65 averaged 63.50 in 2005-2006; 64.12 in 2007-2008 and 65.90 in2009-2010. In 2011-2012, the score was 68.29 showing gradual improvement. The better eating score is credited to changes such as decreased intakes of trans-fats, red meat and sugary drinks. The foods that rated lowest in intake were whole grains and vegetables. Sodium also received a low rating.

Two large scale studies were reported in 2014 showing diet quality and adherence to the Dietary Guidelines by older adults. An Australian study of participants followed for 5 and 10 years, a higher diet quality (high intake of fruits, vegetables, whole grains and fish) was associated with a better quality of life and functional ability. (2) In the second study, over a thousand older adults participated in a "Cardiovascular Health of Seniors and Built Environment Study"(3). Eating scores were slightly higher for women than men. Daily energy intakes were less than recommended but both men and women consumed adequate amounts of carbohydrate and protein and were in the upper range for percentage of energy from total fat, saturated fat, trans-fat and added sugar. Both exceeded sodium intake recommendations and had inadequate intakes of fiber, calcium, magnesium, potassium, zinc, folate, vitamins A, B-6, C, D and E. The poor showing for many nutrients indicate a continued need for more education for the public.

The *National Health and Nutrition Examination Survey (NHANES)* is a program designed to assess the health and nutritional status of U.S. persons.(4) The yearly program combines interviews and physical examinations. It is a major program of the National Center for Health Statistics of the Centers for Disease Control that was begun in the 1960's. The program uses a series of surveys focusing on different population groups or health topics and examines a nationally representative sample of about 5000 persons a year.

The survey includes demographic, socioeconomic, dietary and health-related questions as well as medical, dental and physiologic measurements. The findings help determine the prevalence of major diseases and risk factors for diseases and assessments of nutritional status and its association with health promotion and disease prevention. With this comprehensive amount of information, health knowledge for the nation is greatly expanded.

Healthy People 2020

The Department of Health and Human Services issues health goals for the United States each ten years. (5) The goals represent concerted efforts to improve the health of all Americans through a combination of programs conducted by multiple groups and driven by the best available evidence and knowledge. There are four overarching goals described as targets to be attained through specific measures designed to show progress during the ten-year effort. The four goals are the following:

1. Attain high quality, longer lives free of preventable diseases, disability, injury and premature death.

2. Achieve health equity, eliminate disparities and improve the health of all groups.
3. Create social and physical environments that promote good health for all.
4. Promote quality of life, healthy development, and healthy behaviors across all life stages.

The goals further designate 26 Health Indicators organized under 12 "leading health indicators". One of the 12 topics is "Nutrition, Physical Activity and Obesity" with a list of specific expected targets under each topic. At the approximate halfway point between 2010 and 2020, the number of adults meeting physical activity and muscle-strengthening guidelines exceeded the target set earlier. Obesity rates increased however among both adults and children as did the mean daily intake of total vegetables, which is one of the designated goals.

Summary

The Dietary Guidelines and Healthy People 2020 both give direction to the efforts to improve the health of all U.S. persons at all ages. While the Dietary Guidelines focus on food, nutrition and good eating habits, the Healthy People are much broader goals covering almost all aspects of physical and mental health with targets for achievement.

References

1. www.cnnp.usda.gov
2. Gopinath B, Russell J, Flood VN, Burlutsky G, Mitchell P. Adherence to Dietary Guidelines Positively Affects Quality of Life and Functional Status of Older Adults. J Acad Nutr Diet 2014;114(2):220-229.
3. Delerlein AL, Marland KB, Scanlin K, Wong S. Spark A. Diet Quality of Urban Older Adults Age 60 to 99 years. "The Cardiovascular Health of Seniors and Built Environment Study." J Acad Nutr Diet 2014;114(2):279-287.
4. www.nhanes.cdc.gov
5. www.healthypeople.hhs.gov

Chapter 11

Food and Nutrition Priorities at Spanish Cove

The Spanish Cove Retirement Center at Yukon, Oklahoma, is a Continuing Care Community in existence for 40 years. During that time, it has established a reputation as a leading facility in the state with continued emphasis on optimal quality of life for its residents. This extends to all levels of care—independent living, assisted living, and skilled nursing care.

An important part of living arrangements integral to resident health and overall satisfaction is the food service. This is accomplished through close attention to both food preparation and food service with special menus for holidays and other events. A central food preparation area prepares meals for independent-living residents who are served in a central dining room and in dining areas located in the assisted living and nursing center areas. Dining areas are attractively furnished and decorated with seasonal themes.

Extensive food selection is offered, generally with a choice of three or more entrees, several vegetables, a wide variety of salads and several dessert choices. A side bar offering typical dishes—for example, American, Mexican, "potato", and "pizza" bars are provided on certain week days. In addition, two entrees or salads are offered each week as specialty health items lower in calories, salt and sugar. Sugar-free desserts, fruit, ice cream and yogurt are always available for dessert. On-order sandwiches and salads are also prepared when requested.

Several meal plans are available to independent residents, i.e., 30, 20 or other meals a month. Changes may be made at any time as residents choose.

The food service staff prepares meals based on a five-week cycle. The menus are printed and provided residents weekly. In addition to the dining room meal service, carry-out meals may be ordered which are then delivered to individual apartments. This is a greatly-appreciated service during bad weather or illness as the dining facilities are in a separate building from the apartments and homes.

Another special feature is a once-a –month birthday dinner celebration for all residents having birthdays that particular month. Special holiday meals are always offered, with families and guests welcomed, and with special holiday themes and decorations.

Food Choices

Food selections by residents follow typical patterns for older age groups. Beef pot roast, shrimp and chicken breast are among the most-often chosen meat items. Baked potatoes, green beans, corn and carrots are the most popular vegetables. Pizzas are universally popular and are offered once weekly. Fruit cobblers, pies and ice cream are the preferred dessert items.

In general, residents appear to eat healthfully. This may well be the outcome of the types of food offered and the avoidance of "fast" or highly processed food. Healthful food choices may also be a significant factor in the relative overall good health and general fitness of residents.

Resident Food Committee

A food committee of residents is appointed each year by the Town Hall Council, the resident's organization that conducts programs and interacts with the administration. The committee conducts a yearly survey of all residents regarding the food and food service. The results are shared with the food service director and he, in turn, reports back to the entire group regarding the comments and suggestions that were submitted including any actions to be taken.

Nutrition Education

Nutrition and nutrition education is an important part of the overall dietary management for residents at Spanish Cove. Information is provided on the menus about items that are "heart-healthy", i.e., lower in fat, sodium and calories. In addition, a complete listing of the nutrient content of menu items is available. A nutritionist oversees food intakes among residents in assisted and nursing areas with personal attention in regard to nutritional intakes as may be needed by individuals. Assistance is provided for persons who need diabetic or modified texture diets.

Once a month, a power point presentation on topics in nutrition, health and aging issues is presented by a PhD nutritionist who is a former Oklahoma State University professor in nutrition. The sessions feature a wide range of topics in all areas of nutrition, mental and physical health issues, aging and chronic diseases. Educational handouts are provided and, when applicable, snacks or food items pertinent to the subject of the day are provided.

As a follow-up to the lectures, at one point residents were offered an opportunity to have a four- week record of their self-reported food intake analyzed for nutrient content by the nutritionist. Six women and one man completed the records. Those who followed through could be described as ones generally making good food choices and who were willing to reveal their choices. The analyses were given each individual. In general, calorie intakes were low—about two-thirds of the recommended levels of intake. Protein, fat and vitamin B 12 were at or slightly above recommended intakes while calcium and iron intakes were low. The calorie intake may be questionable as these particular residents do exercise and can be said to be in reasonably good health. The results, however, are in line with other studies that have been reported about the nutrient intakes of older adults. They may or may not reflect the overall nutritional intakes of residents because it was such a small number of residents. A longer study with more participants who keep records of their food intake would give a more complete picture of the nutritional status of Spanish Cove residents.

Summary

Food preparation and food service at Spanish Cove is a very important part of the goal of providing the best possible health outcomes for the residents. Nutritious, attractive and appetizing food choices help meet this goal as do nutrition and health lectures that provide up-to-date information for help in making good food choices and thus optimizing overall health.

The Chapter 12
Healthy People Living Longer Better

"Healthy People 2020" is a nationwide effort by the Department of Health and Human Services to improve the health of all Americans. Goals to be achieved are set each ten-year period, currently 2010-2020, and progress monitored toward reaching the goals. The four overarching goals are identified in Chapter 10.

In 2010, when the current set of goals were published, a particular category—obesity—had increased among adults aged 20 and older during the preceding period and this was one of the areas of health stressed in the new goals. The good news was that adults meeting the physical activity and muscle-strengthening guidelines increased by about 13 percent from earlier years but little change in dietary habits was noted.

Leading Health Indicators

Twelve "Leading Health Indicators" are identified out of 26 overall categories of health, each with multiple objectives. Among the twelve , the ones most applicable to the older adult population from a physical and mental standpoint and to Spanish Cove residents are:

1. Access to health services
2. Clinical preventive services
3. Mental health
4. Nutrition, Physical Activity and Obesity
5. Oral health

Meeting the Goals

At Spanish Cove, the management team has from the beginning established the facility as one focused on providing the best possible attention and care for residents. To that end, health goals at national, state and local levels are observed and followed. In this review of ways that Spanish Cove meets the five above-stated Health Indicators, each is discussed with specific activities in effect.

Access to Health Services: Residents have access through insurance plans, primarily Medicare and secondary plans. A medical clinic is located on the campus open to all residents for immediate care. As well, most residents have access to private physicians for general and specialty care. Residents in assisted and nursing care are provided full-time nursing care and physical therapy services. Those in independent living residences have access to home nursing care as needed for lesser health problems and care following hospitalizations or surgery.

Clinical Preventive Services: Through home nursing care, monitoring of high blood pressure, flu and pneumonococcal inoculations, and help with diabetes management are examples of care provided. Each resident's needs are met through direct assistance, educational programs and healthful activities.

Mental Health: This assistance is addressed in several way. Educational talks stress brain and heart healthy dietary habits as ways of maintaining mental health. Physical activity, which is readily available, is a strong facilitator of mental health. At admission, residents are asked to complete the mini-mental test. As a part of the physical fitness tests described earlier, a mental component is included along with the other tests. Spanish Cove also participates in a music and memory program as well as utilizes other evidence-based tools in working with residents experiencing dementia.

Nutrition, Physical Activity and Obesity: This goal stresses attainment of physical exercise and muscle-strengthening, treatment of obesity and nutritional health. A sizeable number of independent-living residents (and some residents in assisted living) at Spanish Cove participate in one or more of the physical activity programs available. The fitness department also owns an *Inbody* machine for measurement of total body composition (fat and lean body mass) as well as all standard exercise equipment for use by individuals. Treatment of obesity among residents occurs through educational programs and demonstrations as well as through low calorie menu options. A recent weight-loss competition among staff resulted in some positive results regarding lost weight.

Oral Health: This is essentially an individual responsibility except when poor dental health leads to difficulty in chewing or when changes in taste and smell lead to poor appetite and lowered food intake. These types of problems are often associated with malnutrition, lowered disease resistance and generally poor health.

Looking to the Future

Through collaborative studies with the University of Central Oklahoma and Oklahoma State University in fitness testing of residents, the Spanish Cove administration is convinced that such continued cooperative efforts can significantly demonstrate the value of research and special studies in the care of older adults. The studies can be facilitated by linking with universities, state agencies or other entities such as Foundations or private companies who have interests in areas of study such as gerontology, health promotion, biosytems engineering, nutrition, management, sociology, physical recreation, etc. Funded research with University faculty or short-term studies to fulfill specific objectives in areas of need are examples of joint efforts.

Several specific areas of possible study are suggested as follows:

- Health status. Example: persons with diabetes well controlled and not well controlled; practices and knowledge regarding complications, care etc.
- Health indicators. Dr. visits, physical therapy received, self-treatments, use of supplements, etc.
- Drugs and medication usage
- Degree of independence such as average length of time

in independent living and the extent of help needed in activities of daily living.

- Fitness and physical health studies: types, numbers participating, status of participants
- Results of participation in physical activities over time in regard to stamina, strength, frailty, weight, etc.
- Nutritional status studies focusing on usual dietary intakes, intake of specific nutrients related to health problems, etc.
- Food intake studies to show food patterns, likes and dislikes, knowledge and use of food labeling
- Nutrition in prevention, treatment and management of chronic diseases: knowledge, practices etc.
- Post-retirement activities and continuing education opportunities
- Social interactions
- Educational and recreational activities
- Use of technology
- Resident involvement in facility administration
- Staffing and volunteerism

Study Benefits

As studies are initiated and conducted, it is important that data is collected that correlates with prevention, treatment and management of chronic disease conditions. It is estimated that about 80 percent of all Medicare spending is attributable to 15 percent of the Medicare population who have serious or multiple chronic conditions and chronic conditions are a huge driver of health care costs. The Centers for Disease Control indicates that 86 percent of the nation's 2.7 trillion annual health care expenditures are for people with chronic and mental health conditions. (1) Heart disease and cancer accounted for almost half of all deaths in 2014 while obesity, diabetes and arthritis are all disabling conditions requiring extensive health care. It is obvious that extensive efforts are needed in order to curb health risk behaviors, prevent the onset of chronic conditions and lower costs of treatment.

Summary

The Federal Government issues health goals each ten-year period for the country. The goals provide a guide for implementing programs and activities that lead to better health for all. As a premier retirement community in Oklahoma, Spanish Cove conducts a variety of successful programs for residents for health maintenance and improvement. Further studies and research in collaboration with universities, state agencies, foundations or private enterprises would benefit and enhance these efforts.

References

1. www.cdc.gov.nchs/data/hus15

Appendix A

American College of Sports Medicine Guidelines for Physical Activity in Adults over age 65 (or Adults with Chronic Conditions, such as arthritis).

AEROBIC ACTMTY

Frequency: 3-5 times per week

Intensity: Moderate intensity exercise on a scale of 1-10 (1 feeling extremely easy and 10 feeling extremely fatigued), you should feel like a 6. You should be able to hold a conversation while working out.

Time: 20-30 minutes per day

Type: Aerobic (walking, jogging, elliptical machine , biking, etc.)

Enjoyment: Enjoyable aerobic activities

All aerobic activity should consist of three parts

Warm Up - 5-10 minutes of stretching and activity at 50% of intensity

Endurance- At least 20-30 minutes at 60-90% of Maximum Heart Rate

Cool Down - 5-10 minutes of stretching and activity at 50% intensity

STRENGTH ACTIVITY

Frequency: 2 to 3 times per week

Repetitions: 10-15 per set

Sets: 2-3 per exercise

Intensity: Do 10-15 reps with proper form. If you can perform over 15 reps, increase the weight by 2 pounds . If you can't perform more than 10, decrease the weight by 2 pounds

Strength Training Guidelines

Briefly warm-up prior to EACH exercise.

Do at least one set of 10-15 repetitions of each exercise to the point of fatigue.

Increase resistance when 10-15 repetitions can be completed

using proper form. Typically use increments of 2-5% of weight or 2-5 pounds.

Strength train at least two days per week. Allow 48 hours of rest between workouts.

Perform both the lifting and lowering phases of the exercise in a slow and controlled manner. Remember, never sacrifice form for weight.

Perform exercises through a full range of motion.

Maintain a normal breathing pattern throughout the exercise.

If possible, exercise with a friend. Partners can provide encouragement and assistance.

Flexibility -

Find 10 minutes to stretch each major musc le /tendons after you exercise. Hold each stretch 10-30 seconds. Repeat 3 to 4 times. Flexibility will allow you to perform everyday activities with less pain and more ease.

ACTIVITY PLAN

Consult your physician about developing an activity plan that takes into account your specific therapeutic needs and health risks .

GENERAL GUIDELINES

Strength Training is very important for all adults, but especially in older adults. Strength Training prevents loss of bone density and loss of muscle mass.

Physical activity helps promote circulation and mobility and will enhance your functionality, that is , your ability to perform everyday tasks.

Appendix B

The MIND Diet Plan

MIND: "Mediterranean-DASH Intervention for Neurodegenerative Delay"

Green leafy vegetables (example spinach, kale, green lettuce, other greens).
At least one serving per day.

Other vegetables:
At least one other vegetable a day.

Whole grains:
Three or more servings a day

Beans (kidney, white, soy, black, dry lima etc.):
At least 3 servings a week

Nuts (avoid salt and sugared nuts):
Five one-ounce servings a week

Berries (all kinds, especially blueberries, fresh or frozen)
Two or more servings a week

Fish (especially oily fish like salmon, trout etc. not fried or breaded)
Once a week

Poultry (chicken, turkey-- not fried)
Two servings a week

Olive oil as the primary cooking oil.

Wine if desired. One glass a day

Red Meat:
Less than four servings a week

Butter and margarine:
One tablespoon or less per day

Cheese
Less than one serving a week

Pastries and sweets
Less than five servings a week

Fried or fast food
Less than one serving a week

Water, tea, coffee
8 glasses per day

Appendix C

DASH Eating Plan

Food Group	Daily Servings	Serving Sizes
Grains (whole grains recommended)	6-8	1 slice bread 1 oz dry cereal 1/2 cup cooked rice, pasta, or cereal
Vegetables	4-5	1 cup raw leafy vegetable 1/2 cup cut raw or cooked vegetable 1/2 cup vegetable juice
Fruits	4-5	1 medium fruit 1/4 cup dried fruit 1/2 cup fresh, frozen, or canned fruit 1/2 cup fruit juice
Fat-free or low-fat milk and milk products	2-3	1 cup milk or yogurt 1 1/2 oz cheese
Lean meats, poultry, and fish	6 or less	1 oz cooked meats, poultry. or fish 1 egg**
Nuts, seeds, and legumes	4-5 per week	1/3 cup or 11/2 oz nuts 2 Tbsp peanut butter 2 Tbsp or 1/3 oz seeds 1/2 cup cooked legumes (dry beans and peas)
Fats and oils	2-3	1 tsp soft margarine 1 tsp vegetable oil 1 Tbsp mayonnaise 2 Tbsp salad dressing
Sweets and added sugars	5 or less per week	1 Tbsp sugar 1 Tbsp jelly or jam 1/3 cup sorbet, gelatin 1 cup lemonade

Source: "Your Guide to Lowering Your Blood Pressure with DASH."
USDHHS Nat. Institute of Health, National Heart, Lung, and Blood
Institute.

Appendix D

Mediterranean Diet Plan at 2000 Calorie Level

FOOD	SERVING AMOUNT
Dark green vegetables	1 ½ cups per week
Red and orange vegetables	5 ½ cups per week
Legumes (beans and peas)	1 ½ cups per week
Starchy vegetables	5 cups per week
Other vegetables	5 cups per week
Fruits	2 ½ cups per week
Grains	6 ounces per week
Whole grains	3 ounces per day
Refined grains	3 ounces per day
Seafood	15 ounces per week
Meat, poultry, eggs	6 ounces per week
Nuts, seeds, soy products	5 ounces per week
Oils	5 ½ ounces per week
Other calorie sources	26

Appendix E

U.S. Department of Agriculture (USDA) Food Plans

Daily Amount of Food From Each Group

Food	1800 Calories	2000 Calories	2200 Calories
Fruits	1 ½ cups	2 cups	2 cups
Vegetables	2 ½ cups	2 ½ cups	2 cups
Grains	6 ounces	6 ounces	8 ounces
Prot ein foods	5 ounces	5 ½ ounces	6 ounces
Dairy	3 cups	3 cups	3 cups
Oils	1 ounce	1 ounce	1 ounce
Extra calories	160	260	265

Appendix F

Body Mass Index Table

Body Weight (pounds)

Height (inches)	Normal						Overweight					Obese										Extreme Obesity														
BMI	19	20	21	22	23	24	25	26	27	28	29	30	31	32	33	34	35	36	37	38	39	40	41	42	43	44	45	46	47	48	49	50	51	52	53	54
58	91	96	100	105	110	115	119	124	129	134	138	143	148	153	158	162	167	172	177	181	186	191	196	201	205	210	215	220	224	229	234	239	244	248	253	258
59	94	99	104	109	114	119	124	128	133	138	143	148	153	158	163	168	173	178	183	188	193	198	203	208	212	217	222	227	232	237	242	247	252	257	262	267
60	97	102	107	112	118	123	128	133	138	143	148	153	158	163	168	174	179	184	189	194	199	204	209	215	220	225	230	235	240	245	250	255	261	266	271	276
61	100	106	111	116	122	127	132	137	143	148	153	158	164	169	174	180	185	190	195	201	206	211	217	222	227	232	238	243	248	254	259	264	269	275	280	285
62	104	109	115	120	126	131	136	142	147	153	158	164	169	175	180	186	191	196	202	207	213	218	224	229	235	240	246	251	256	262	267	273	278	284	289	295
63	107	113	118	124	130	135	141	146	152	158	163	169	175	180	186	191	197	203	208	214	220	225	231	237	242	248	254	259	265	270	278	282	287	293	299	304
64	110	116	122	128	134	140	145	151	157	163	169	174	180	186	192	197	204	209	215	221	227	232	238	244	250	256	262	267	273	279	285	291	296	302	308	314
65	114	120	126	132	138	144	150	156	162	168	174	180	186	192	198	204	210	216	222	228	234	240	246	252	258	264	270	276	282	288	294	300	306	312	318	324
66	118	124	130	136	142	148	155	161	167	173	179	186	192	198	204	210	216	223	229	235	241	247	253	260	266	272	278	284	291	297	303	309	315	322	328	334
67	121	127	134	140	146	153	159	166	172	178	185	191	198	204	211	217	223	230	236	242	249	255	261	268	274	280	287	293	299	306	312	319	325	331	338	344
68	125	131	138	144	151	158	164	171	177	184	190	197	203	210	216	223	230	236	243	249	256	262	269	276	282	289	295	302	308	315	322	328	335	341	348	354
69	128	135	142	149	155	162	169	176	182	189	196	203	209	216	223	230	236	243	250	257	263	270	277	284	291	297	304	311	318	324	331	338	345	351	358	365
70	132	139	146	153	160	167	174	181	188	195	202	209	216	222	229	236	243	250	257	264	271	278	285	292	299	306	313	320	327	334	341	348	355	362	369	376
71	136	143	150	157	165	172	179	186	193	200	208	215	222	229	236	243	250	257	265	272	279	286	293	301	308	315	322	329	338	343	351	358	365	372	379	386
72	140	147	154	162	169	177	184	191	199	206	213	221	228	235	242	250	258	265	272	279	287	294	302	309	316	324	331	338	346	353	361	368	375	383	390	397
73	144	151	159	166	174	182	189	197	204	212	219	227	235	242	250	257	265	272	280	288	295	302	310	318	325	333	340	348	355	363	371	378	386	393	401	408
74	148	155	163	171	179	186	194	202	210	218	225	233	241	249	256	264	272	280	287	295	303	311	319	326	334	342	350	358	365	373	381	389	396	404	412	420
75	152	160	168	176	184	192	200	208	216	224	232	240	248	256	264	272	279	287	295	303	311	319	327	335	343	351	359	367	375	383	391	399	407	415	423	431
76	156	164	172	180	189	197	205	213	221	230	238	246	254	263	271	279	287	295	304	312	320	328	336	344	353	361	369	377	385	394	402	410	418	426	435	443

Source: Adapted from *Clinical Guidelines on the Identification, Evaluation, and Treatment of Overweight and Obesity in Adults: The Evidence Report.*

Appendix G

*Dietary Reference Intakes (DRI) for Age 70
Plus Male and Female*

CALORIES	MALE	FEMALE
Sedentary	2000	1600
Moderately active	2200	1800
Active	2600	2000
PROTEIN, g	56	46
FAT, g	20-35% of calories (male and female)	
CARBOHYDRATE, g	45-65% of calories (male and female)	
VITAMIN A, ug	900	700
THIAMIN, mg	1.1	90
RIBOFLAVIN, mg	1.3	1.1
NIACIN, mg	16	14
VITAMIN B-6, mg	1.7	1.5
FOLATE, ug	400	400
VITAMIN B-12, ug	2.4	2.4
VITAMIN C, mg	90	75
VITAMIN D, ug	15	15
VITAMIN E, mg	15	15
CALCIUM, mg	1200	1200
IRON, mg	8.0	8.0

PHOSPHORUS, mg	700	700
SELENIUM, ug	55	55
MAGNESIUM, mg	420	420
ZINC, mg	11	8,0
POTASSIUM, g	4.7	4.7
SODIUM, g	1.2	1.2
FIBER, g	30	2.1

www.ingramcontent.com/pod-product-compliance
Lightning Source LLC
Chambersburg PA
CBHW052140270326
41930CB00012B/2965

9 781581 073157